SUPER EASY
ANTI-INFLAMMATORY
DIET

A Beginner's Cookbook to Reduce Inflammation, Balance Gut Health, and Regulate Your Immune System. Includes a 28-Day Meal Plan

TABLE OF CONTENT

Introduction

Inflammation is a natural immune response, a signal that your body is fighting against something that could harm it, such as infections, injuries, and toxins. However, when inflammation becomes chronic, it can lead to a host of health problems, including heart disease, diabetes, cancer, and arthritis. Understanding the dual nature of inflammation—as both a necessary defense mechanism and a potential health threat—is crucial in navigating the complexities of our body's response to harm.

The modern diet, rich in processed foods, sugars, and unhealthy fats, plays a significant role in promoting chronic inflammation. Conversely, a diet focused on whole, nutrient-dense foods can help reduce inflammation. This is where the anti-inflammatory diet comes into play. It is not a diet in the traditional sense of weight loss but a way of eating that supports your body's health and well-being. By emphasizing foods rich in antioxidants, phytochemicals, and omega-3 fatty acids, the anti-inflammatory diet aims to balance gut health, regulate the immune system, and reduce the chronic inflammation that contributes to disease.

The anti-inflammatory diet is grounded in the understanding that food is medicine. What we eat can have a profound effect on our body's inflammatory processes. This diet encourages the consumption of fruits, vegetables, whole grains, lean protein, and healthy fats, all of which contribute to reducing inflammation. It also advises limiting intake of processed foods, red meats, and foods high in added sugars and saturated fats.

This book, "Super Easy Anti-Inflammatory Diet Cookbook," is designed to make the principles of the anti-inflammatory diet accessible and practical for everyday life. Whether you are new to the concept of anti-inflammatory eating or looking to expand your repertoire of healthful recipes, this book offers a comprehensive guide to reducing inflammation through diet. With a focus on simple, quick-to-prepare dishes made with readily available ingredients, it aims to support your journey towards a healthier, more balanced diet.

The recipes and insights provided in this book are more than just a collection of meals; they are a testament to the power of food to heal and nourish our bodies. By making informed choices about what we eat, we can take control of our health and well-being. The anti-inflammatory diet is not about restriction but about embracing a wide variety of delicious, healthful foods that not only taste good but also do good for our bodies.

Inflammation and You

Inflammation is a term that often carries a negative connotation, primarily due to its association with various chronic diseases. However, it's important to recognize that inflammation is fundamentally a protective response, initiated by the body's immune system to remove harmful stimuli and initiate the healing process. The complexity of inflammation lies in its dual nature: it is both beneficial in acute scenarios and potentially harmful when it becomes chronic.

Acute inflammation is the body's immediate response to injury or infection, characterized by redness, heat, swelling, and pain. This type of inflammation is short-lived, lasting only a few days. It plays a crucial role in protecting and healing the body. For instance, if you cut your finger, the acute inflammatory response helps to eliminate invading bacteria and starts the healing process.

In contrast, chronic inflammation is a prolonged inflammatory response that can last for months or even years. Unlike acute inflammation, which is a necessary part of the healing process, chronic inflammation can be detrimental to health. It arises when the immune system continuously produces inflammatory cells even in the absence of external threats. This persistent state of alert can lead to the damage of healthy cells, tissues, and organs, and is linked to a range of chronic conditions, including heart disease, diabetes, cancer, and autoimmune diseases.

The connection between diet and inflammation is significant and complex. Certain foods, such as processed meats, refined carbs, and sugary beverages, can exacerbate inflammatory responses in the body. These foods can trigger the immune system to produce an excessive number of inflammatory cells, leading to chronic inflammation. On the other hand, a diet rich in whole, nutrient-dense foods like fruits, vegetables, whole grains, and fatty fish can help reduce inflammation. These foods contain antioxidants, phytochemicals, and omega-3 fatty acids, which have been shown to have anti-inflammatory effects.

Understanding the types of inflammation and the impact of diet on inflammatory responses is crucial for adopting an anti-inflammatory diet. This diet focuses on consuming foods that support the body's natural ability to heal and protect against disease. By making informed dietary choices, individuals can significantly influence their body's inflammatory processes, promoting overall health and well-being.

The anti-inflammatory diet is not about strict restrictions or eliminating entire food groups but about creating a balanced, nutrient-rich eating pattern that supports the body's immune system and reduces the risk of chronic inflammation. It emphasizes the importance of quality over quantity, encouraging the consumption of foods that are as close to their natural state as possible.

Defining Inflammation: Acute vs. Chronic

Inflammation is the body's innate mechanism for defending itself against harm, whether from an invading pathogen, an injury, or a toxin. This response is crucial for survival, initiating the healing process by mobilizing the immune system to fight off the offending agent and begin repairs. Acute inflammation is characterized by four cardinal signs: redness, heat, swelling, and pain. These symptoms are the result of the immune system's efforts to eliminate the harmful stimuli and facilitate tissue recovery. For example, the redness and heat are due to increased blood flow to the affected area, bringing with it immune cells to combat the invaders and initiate healing. Swelling occurs as fluids accumulate, and pain serves as a signal to the body that something is wrong, often prompting the individual to take action to protect the area.

Contrastingly, chronic inflammation represents a prolonged, often low-grade immune response that fails to resolve. Unlike the acute response, which is immediate and generally beneficial, chronic inflammation can be insidious, persisting without a clear cause or after the initial threat has been eliminated. Over time, this type of inflammation can lead to the degradation of healthy tissues and organs, subtly undermining physiological functions and contributing to the development of numerous chronic diseases. The mechanisms behind chronic inflammation are complex, involving a persistent activation of the immune system that leads to tissue damage and alterations in cellular processes. This can be triggered by various factors, including persistent infections, exposure to environmental toxins, and, notably, lifestyle factors such as diet.

The role of diet in inflammation is profound. Certain foods, particularly those high in refined sugars, saturated fats, and trans fats, can exacerbate inflammatory processes, contributing to the chronic inflammation associated with many modern diseases. These dietary components can stimulate the immune system in an adverse way, leading to an overproduction of inflammatory cells and signaling molecules that perpetuate inflammation. Conversely, a diet rich in whole foods, such as fruits, vegetables, whole grains, and omega-3 fatty acids, can help modulate the body's inflammatory response. These foods contain compounds that can reduce inflammation, including antioxidants that neutralize free radicals and other substances that can dampen the production of pro-inflammatory molecules.

Understanding the distinction between acute and chronic inflammation is essential for recognizing the impact of lifestyle choices on health. While acute inflammation is a necessary and protective response to immediate threats, chronic inflammation can be a silent adversary, contributing to the development of disease under the radar. By making informed dietary choices, individuals have the power to influence their inflammatory status, potentially reducing their risk of chronic disease and improving their overall health and well-being. This knowledge forms the foundation for adopting an anti-inflammatory diet, emphasizing the importance of dietary patterns that support the body's natural defenses and promote long-term health.

The Impact of Inflammation on Health and Well-being

Chronic inflammation acts as a silent catalyst for a myriad of health issues, subtly undermining the body's systems and contributing to the onset and progression of various diseases. It is a key player in the development of arthritis, where it causes painful swelling and stiffness in the joints, significantly impairing mobility and quality of life. In the realm of cardiovascular health, chronic inflammation is a recognized risk factor for heart disease, contributing to plaque buildup in the arteries, which can lead to heart attacks and strokes. Furthermore, it plays a significant role in metabolic disorders, including diabetes, by affecting insulin sensitivity and glucose metabolism, thereby disrupting the body's ability to manage blood sugar levels effectively.

The link between chronic inflammation and cancer is also well-documented, with inflammation both promoting the initiation and aiding the progression of various cancers by creating an environment conducive to tumor growth and spread. Additionally, neurological disorders such as Alzheimer's disease have been associated with chronic inflammatory processes, suggesting that inflammation may contribute to neurodegeneration and cognitive decline.

Beyond these direct associations with specific diseases, chronic inflammation exerts a more insidious influence on general health and well-being. It is often accompanied by less obvious signs that can be easily overlooked or attributed to other causes. Fatigue is a common symptom, where individuals experience a pervasive sense of tiredness and lack of energy that is not relieved by rest. Digestive problems, including irregular bowel movements, bloating, and discomfort, can also indicate an underlying inflammatory response. Moreover, unexplained aches and pains, not linked to acute injury or exercise, may be manifestations of systemic inflammation affecting various parts of the body.

These subtler signs of chronic inflammation underscore the importance of awareness and proactive management through lifestyle choices, particularly diet. By recognizing the potential health effects of prolonged inflammation and its less obvious manifestations, individuals can take informed steps towards mitigating its impact. Adopting an anti-inflammatory diet, rich in whole foods and nutrients that support the body's natural anti-inflammatory processes, offers a practical approach to reducing chronic inflammation and promoting overall health and well-being.

How Your Diet Influences Inflammatory Responses

Diet plays a pivotal role in influencing inflammatory responses within the body. Certain foods, particularly those that are heavily processed, high in sugars, trans fats, and specific types of oils, can significantly exacerbate inflammation. These pro-inflammatory foods trigger a cascade of reactions in the body that can lead to an increase in inflammatory markers. For instance, processed foods often contain additives and preservatives that can disrupt the body's natural inflammatory processes. Similarly, high levels of sugars and trans fats in the diet can lead to an imbalance in the body's natural mechanisms for regulating inflammation, contributing to chronic inflammatory conditions.

Conversely, anti-inflammatory foods are those that support the body's natural ability to combat inflammation. These foods are rich in antioxidants, fibers, and omega-3 fatty acids, all of which play crucial roles in modulating inflammatory responses. Antioxidants, found abundantly in fruits and vegetables, help neutralize free radicals, thereby reducing oxidative stress and inflammation. Fibers, particularly those from whole grains and legumes, support gut health, which is closely linked to inflammation. A healthy gut microbiota can influence systemic inflammation positively. Omega-3 fatty acids, found in fatty fish, flaxseeds, and walnuts, are known for their anti-inflammatory properties. They help reduce the production of inflammatory eicosanoids and cytokines, molecules that play key roles in the inflammatory process.

The importance of dietary patterns over individual foods cannot be overstated. While incorporating specific anti-inflammatory foods into one's diet is beneficial, adopting a comprehensive dietary pattern that emphasizes these foods is more effective in reducing inflammation. The Mediterranean diet is a prime example of such a pattern. Characterized by a high intake of fruits, vegetables, whole grains, olive oil, fish, and moderate wine consumption, the Mediterranean diet has been extensively studied and shown to reduce markers of inflammation. Its emphasis on whole, unprocessed foods rich in anti-inflammatory nutrients supports the body's natural defenses against inflammation.

Sustainable dietary habits, like those promoted by the Mediterranean diet, offer a holistic approach to managing inflammation through diet. By focusing on a diverse intake of nutrient-dense foods and minimizing the consumption of processed foods, sugars, and unhealthy fats, individuals can significantly influence their inflammatory status. This approach not only aids in reducing inflammation but also supports overall health and well-being, highlighting the critical role of diet in managing inflammation and preventing related chronic diseases. Adopting such dietary patterns can be a powerful strategy for enhancing one's health, demonstrating the profound impact of diet on inflammatory responses.

The Science of Anti-Inflammatory Eating

The nutritional science behind the anti-inflammatory diet reveals a fascinating interplay between the foods we consume and our body's inflammatory responses. Central to this diet are antioxidants, phytochemicals, and omega-3 fatty acids, each playing a unique role in mitigating inflammation and fostering overall health.

Antioxidants are compounds that protect the body from oxidative stress, a condition that occurs when there are too many free radicals—unstable molecules that can damage cells—relative to antioxidants. This imbalance leads to oxidative stress, which plays a pivotal role in the development of chronic inflammation and related diseases. Foods rich in antioxidants, such as berries, nuts, and green leafy vegetables, supply the body with the means to neutralize free radicals, thereby reducing oxidative stress and inflammation.

Phytochemicals, naturally occurring compounds found in plants, offer another layer of protection against inflammation. These substances, which include flavonoids, carotenoids, and sulforaphane, have been shown to modulate the immune system and reduce inflammation. They achieve this by inhibiting the production of pro-inflammatory cytokines and enzymes, such as cyclooxygenase-2 (COX-2), which are involved in the inflammatory process. The diverse array of phytochemicals found in fruits, vegetables, whole grains, and legumes underscores the importance of a varied diet rich in plant-based foods.

Omega-3 fatty acids, particularly eicosapentaenoic acid (EPA) and docosahexaenoic acid (DHA), are essential fats that the body cannot produce on its own. Found in fatty fish, flaxseeds, and walnuts, omega-3s are known for their anti-inflammatory properties. They work by reducing the production of molecules and substances linked to inflammation, such as inflammatory eicosanoids and cytokines. Moreover, omega-3 fatty acids can enhance the production of anti-inflammatory compounds, further contributing to their beneficial effects on health.

The link between diet and gut health is another critical aspect of the anti-inflammatory diet. The gut microbiome, consisting of trillions of microorganisms residing in the digestive tract, plays a crucial role in health and disease. A diet high in fiber, particularly from whole grains, fruits, and vegetables, supports a healthy gut microbiome by providing prebiotics—food for beneficial gut bacteria. These beneficial bacteria, in turn, produce short-chain fatty acids (SCFAs) through the fermentation of dietary fiber. SCFAs have been shown to exert anti-inflammatory effects, highlighting the importance of diet in maintaining gut health and reducing inflammation.

In addition to fiber, the consumption of fermented foods rich in probiotics, such as yogurt, kefir, and sauerkraut, can further support gut health by enhancing the diversity and function of the gut microbiome. A healthy gut microbiome is associated with reduced systemic inflammation and a lower risk of chronic diseases, emphasizing the interconnectedness of diet, gut health, and inflammation.

Nutritional Science Behind Anti-Inflammatory Foods

Inflammation, at its core, is the body's response to injury or infection, a fundamental aspect of the immune system's defense mechanism. Acute inflammation is immediate and short-lived, serving as a protective measure to heal the body. Chronic inflammation, however, persists over time, potentially leading to a variety of diseases by damaging healthy cells and tissues. This prolonged state of inflammation is linked to an increased risk of heart disease, diabetes, cancer, and autoimmune conditions, among others. The transition from acute to chronic inflammation underscores the importance of managing inflammatory responses to maintain health.

The biochemical mechanisms through which anti-inflammatory foods exert their effects are complex and multifaceted. These foods contain compounds that can directly influence the body's inflammatory pathways. For instance, they can suppress the production of pro-inflammatory cytokines, which are signaling proteins that promote inflammation. Simultaneously, these foods can enhance the body's production of anti-inflammatory mediators, helping to resolve inflammation and repair tissue. This dual action not only helps to prevent the transition from acute to chronic inflammation but also supports the body's healing processes.

At the heart of managing inflammation through diet is the concept of balance. A balanced diet rich in anti-inflammatory foods can help regulate the body's inflammatory responses. This involves a dietary pattern that emphasizes whole, nutrient-dense foods such as fruits, vegetables, whole grains, lean proteins, and healthy fats. These foods provide a rich source of antioxidants, phytochemicals, and omega-3 fatty acids, all known for their anti-inflammatory properties. Antioxidants help to neutralize free radicals, reducing oxidative stress and inflammation. Phytochemicals, including flavonoids and carotenoids, can modulate immune function and inhibit inflammatory pathways. Omega-3 fatty acids, particularly those found in fatty fish, flaxseeds, and walnuts, have been shown to reduce the production of inflammatory molecules.

The significance of dietary patterns over individual foods cannot be overstated. While incorporating specific anti-inflammatory foods into one's diet is beneficial, adopting an overall dietary pattern that emphasizes these foods is more impactful. Such patterns, including the Mediterranean diet, focus on a holistic approach to eating that supports the body's natural anti-inflammatory processes. This approach not only aids in reducing inflammation but also contributes to overall health and well-being.

The Role of Antioxidants, Phytochemicals, and Omega-3 Fatty Acids

Antioxidants play a pivotal role in combating oxidative stress, a condition characterized by an imbalance between free radicals and antioxidants in your body. Free radicals are unstable molecules that can damage cells, contributing to inflammation and chronic diseases. Antioxidants neutralize these free radicals, thus protecting the body from oxidative stress and inflammation. Foods rich in antioxidants include berries, such as blueberries and strawberries, dark leafy greens like spinach and kale, and nuts, including almonds and walnuts. These foods not only offer a defense against oxidative stress but also provide a variety of nutrients that support overall health.

Phytochemicals are naturally occurring compounds in plants that have been recognized for their role in health and disease prevention. They work through different mechanisms, including the modulation of detoxification enzymes, stimulation of the immune system, and reduction of inflammation. Examples of phytochemicals include flavonoids found in apples and onions, carotenoids present in carrots and tomatoes, and sulforaphane from cruciferous vegetables like broccoli. These compounds can inhibit the production of pro-inflammatory cytokines and enzymes, thereby exerting anti-inflammatory effects. Incorporating a wide range of fruits and vegetables into the diet ensures an adequate intake of these beneficial phytochemicals.

Omega-3 fatty acids are essential fats that the body cannot produce on its own, thus they must be obtained through diet. They are known for their anti-inflammatory properties, which are attributed to their ability to reduce the production of molecules and substances linked to inflammation. There are three main types of omega-3 fatty acids: ALA (alpha-linolenic acid) found in plant sources like flaxseeds and chia seeds, and EPA (eicosapentaenoic acid) and DHA (docosahexaenoic acid), which are primarily found in marine sources such as salmon and mackerel. While all three types are beneficial, EPA and DHA have been more closely associated with reducing inflammation. Balancing omega-3 and omega-6 fatty acids in the diet is crucial, as excessive intake of omega-6s, commonly found in certain vegetable oils, can promote inflammation. Striving for a balance between these fatty acids can help manage inflammation and promote overall health.

Understanding the Gut-Health Connection

The gut microbiome, a complex community of microorganisms residing in the digestive tract, plays a pivotal role in health and disease. It influences not only digestive health but also the immune system and, by extension, systemic inflammation. A diverse microbiome, rich in a variety of beneficial bacteria, can enhance immune function and reduce the risk of chronic inflammation.

Dietary choices have a profound impact on the composition and function of the gut microbiota. Foods that promote a healthy gut are typically rich in fiber, such as fruits, vegetables, and whole grains. These act as prebiotics, feeding beneficial bacteria and encouraging their growth. Fermented foods, like yogurt, kefir, and sauerkraut, are rich in probiotics, live bacteria that add to the diversity of the gut microbiome when consumed. Together, prebiotics and probiotics support a balanced microbiome, which is crucial for maintaining gut integrity and function.

Gut permeability, often referred to as "leaky gut," occurs when the lining of the intestinal wall becomes compromised, allowing substances that should be contained within the gut to leak into the bloodstream. This can trigger an immune response, leading to chronic inflammation and potentially contributing to autoimmune diseases. The integrity of the gut lining is essential for preventing unwanted substances from triggering an immune response, and a healthy, diverse gut microbiome is key to maintaining this barrier.

Anti-inflammatory foods play a significant role in strengthening gut integrity. Omega-3 fatty acids, found in fatty fish, flaxseeds, and walnuts, have been shown to reduce inflammation and may help maintain the gut barrier function. Foods rich in antioxidants and phytochemicals, such as berries, nuts, and green leafy vegetables, can also support gut health by reducing oxidative stress and inflammation, further protecting the gut lining.

Incorporating a variety of whole, nutrient-dense foods into the diet supports a healthy gut microbiome, which in turn can reduce systemic inflammation and lower the risk of chronic diseases. By focusing on a diet rich in fiber, prebiotics, probiotics, and anti-inflammatory foods, individuals can promote gut health, enhance immune function, and contribute to overall well-being.

Navigating the Anti-Inflammatory Diet

Navigating the Anti-Inflammatory Diet requires a strategic approach to food selection and meal planning. This guide is designed to empower you with the knowledge to make informed choices about the foods you eat, the ones you avoid, and how to discern potentially inflammatory ingredients on food labels.

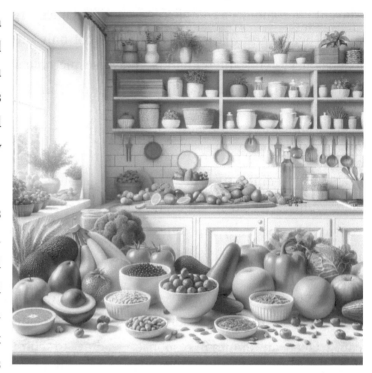

The cornerstone of the anti-inflammatory diet is the emphasis on whole, nutrient-dense foods. These include a variety of colorful fruits and vegetables, whole grains, lean protein sources, and healthy fats. Fruits and vegetables, rich in antioxidants and phytochemicals, combat oxidative stress and inflammation. Whole grains provide fiber, supporting gut health and reducing systemic inflammation. Lean proteins, particularly those from plant sources like legumes and from fish rich in omega-3 fatty acids, contribute to muscle repair and inflammation reduction. Healthy fats, especially those from olive oil, avocados, and nuts, offer anti-inflammatory benefits and support overall health.

Conversely, it's crucial to identify and limit the intake of foods known to promote inflammation. Processed and refined foods, high in added sugars and unhealthy fats, are primary culprits. These foods can disrupt the balance of gut bacteria, leading to increased gut permeability and systemic inflammation. Red and processed meats, high in saturated fats, and certain dairy products can also contribute to inflammatory processes in the body. Additionally, excessive consumption of alcohol and processed snack foods can exacerbate inflammation.

Identifying potentially inflammatory ingredients when shopping is another key skill. Reading labels is essential; look for ingredients like high fructose corn syrup, hydrogenated oils, and artificial additives—these can indicate the presence of pro-inflammatory components. Instead, opt for products with short, recognizable ingredient lists, emphasizing whole foods.

Incorporating anti-inflammatory foods into your diet doesn't have to be a daunting task. Start with simple swaps: replace refined grains with whole grains, choose lean protein sources, and use olive oil instead of butter. Incorporate a variety of fruits and vegetables into every meal to ensure a broad intake of antioxidants and phytochemicals. Experiment with herbs and spices, such as turmeric and ginger, known for their anti-inflammatory properties, to add flavor and health benefits to your meals.

Meal planning can further simplify the transition to an anti-inflammatory diet. Planning your meals and snacks ahead of time ensures that you have the necessary ingredients on hand to prepare nutritious dishes. It also allows you to make mindful choices about your food intake, reducing the likelihood of reaching for processed or fast foods when you're short on time.

Finally, staying hydrated is an often-overlooked aspect of reducing inflammation. Water supports all bodily functions, including the elimination of toxins that can contribute to inflammation. Aim for at least eight glasses of water a day, and consider incorporating anti-inflammatory herbal teas, such as green tea, which offers additional antioxidants.

Core Principles of the Anti-Inflammatory Diet

The anti-inflammatory diet is a strategic approach to eating that prioritizes foods known to reduce inflammation, while minimizing those that can exacerbate it. This diet is not merely about restriction but focuses on enriching the diet with foods that can positively impact health. Its primary goal is to reduce chronic inflammation, a silent contributor to numerous diseases such as heart disease, diabetes, and autoimmune conditions. By adopting this dietary pattern, individuals can significantly lower their risk of these conditions and improve overall well-being.

At the heart of the anti-inflammatory diet are whole foods. These are foods that are consumed as close to their natural state as possible, including a wide variety of fruits and vegetables, whole grains, lean proteins, and healthy fats. These foods are rich in nutrients that combat inflammation, including antioxidants, which protect cells from damage, and phytochemicals, which have various health-promoting properties. Emphasizing whole foods means reducing the intake of processed and refined foods, which often contain unhealthy fats, added sugars, and artificial ingredients that can trigger inflammatory responses.

Balancing the intake of omega-6 and omega-3 fatty acids is another cornerstone of the anti-inflammatory diet. While both types of fats are essential, the typical American diet tends to be disproportionately high in omega-6 fatty acids found in many vegetable oils and processed foods. This imbalance can promote inflammation. Increasing the intake of omega-3 fatty acids, found in fatty fish, flaxseeds, and walnuts, helps restore balance and supports anti-inflammatory processes in the body.

The scientific rationale for the anti-inflammatory diet is grounded in understanding how certain foods influence the body's inflammatory pathways. Antioxidants, for instance, help neutralize free radicals, unstable molecules that can cause oxidative stress and inflammation. Phytochemicals, found in plant-based foods, can modulate the immune system and inhibit enzymes involved in inflammation. Omega-3 fatty acids are known to reduce the production of inflammatory eicosanoids and cytokines. Together, these nutrients work synergistically to reduce inflammation and support the body's natural healing processes.

Foods to Embrace and Those to Avoid

Embracing an anti-inflammatory diet involves a conscious selection of foods that support health and well-being. This dietary approach emphasizes the consumption of whole, nutrient-dense foods known for their anti-inflammatory properties.

Fruits and vegetables are foundational to the anti-inflammatory diet, offering a wide range of antioxidants, vitamins, and minerals that combat inflammation. Berries, such as blueberries and strawberries, are particularly rich in antioxidants, which help neutralize harmful free radicals in the body. Leafy greens, including spinach and kale, provide a wealth of nutrients, including vitamin K, which supports bone health and reduces inflammatory markers.

Nuts and seeds are another important category, offering a good source of healthy fats, protein, and fiber. Almonds, walnuts, and chia seeds, for example, contain omega-3 fatty acids, which are known to reduce inflammation. These foods also provide antioxidants and minerals, such as magnesium, which supports hundreds of biochemical reactions in the body, including those that regulate inflammation.

Whole grains contribute to this diet by providing fiber, which supports digestive health and reduces the risk of chronic diseases. Quinoa, brown rice, and oats are excellent choices that offer a combination of antioxidants, vitamins, and minerals, alongside fiber, helping to modulate the body's inflammatory response.

Fatty fish, such as salmon, mackerel, and sardines, are rich in omega-3 fatty acids, particularly EPA and DHA, which have been extensively studied for their anti-inflammatory effects. Regular consumption of these fish can help reduce the levels of inflammatory markers in the body, supporting cardiovascular health and potentially lowering the risk of chronic diseases.

Healthy oils, especially extra-virgin olive oil, are integral to the anti-inflammatory diet. Olive oil is rich in monounsaturated fats and contains oleocanthal, a compound that has been shown to work similarly to ibuprofen in reducing inflammation.

Conversely, certain foods are known to exacerbate inflammation and should be minimized or avoided. Processed meats, such as sausages and deli meats, contain high levels of saturated fats and additives that can increase inflammation. Refined carbohydrates, found in white bread, pastries, and many processed foods, can lead to spikes in blood sugar and insulin levels, contributing to inflammatory processes.

Overly sugary foods, including soft drinks and candy, are high in fructose, which has been linked to increased uric acid levels and inflammation. Certain vegetable oils, such as corn oil and soybean oil, are high in omega-6 fatty acids. While omega-6s are essential in moderation, an imbalance favoring omega-6s over omega-3s can promote inflammation.

Reading Labels and Identifying Hidden Inflammatory Ingredients

Understanding food labels is a critical skill in adopting an anti-inflammatory diet. Labels provide essential information about the nutritional content of foods, including serving sizes, total calories, and nutrient content. However, they also list ingredients that can be detrimental to your health, many of which are hidden sources of inflammation. Learning to decipher these labels is key to making informed dietary choices that align with anti-inflammatory principles.

Firstly, focus on the serving size and total calories listed on the label. These figures are crucial for understanding how much of a particular nutrient you will consume in a given serving. Misjudging serving sizes can lead to unintentional overconsumption of calories and inflammatory ingredients. Next, examine the nutrient content, paying close attention to dietary fiber, sugars, and types of fats. High fiber content is beneficial, while high levels of sugars and saturated fats are markers of foods that may contribute to inflammation.

Hidden inflammatory ingredients often lurk in the ingredient lists of processed foods. Hydrogenated oils, or trans fats, are known to promote inflammation and are linked to heart disease. They are sometimes listed as "partially hydrogenated oil" in the ingredients. High fructose corn syrup, a common sweetener in processed foods, can trigger inflammation and lead to insulin resistance. Monosodium glutamate (MSG), another additive found in many processed and packaged foods, can also contribute to inflammatory responses, particularly in individuals sensitive to this compound.

When shopping, adopt a strategy that prioritizes fresh produce and minimally processed foods. Stick to the outer aisles of the grocery store, where fresh fruits, vegetables, lean proteins, and dairy products are typically located. Be wary of foods marketed as "health foods" or "natural," as these labels can be misleading. Always check the ingredient list for hidden inflammatory ingredients, even in products that appear to be healthy.

Here are additional tips for smart shopping:

- Choose products with short, recognizable ingredient lists. The fewer the ingredients, the less processed the food is likely to be.

- Look for whole food ingredients at the beginning of the list, as ingredients are listed in order of predominance by weight.

- Be cautious of "sugar-free" or "low-fat" products, as they may contain artificial sweeteners or additives that can contribute to inflammation.

- Opt for products with unsaturated fats from sources like olive oil or nuts, rather than saturated fats or trans fats.

- Consider using a mobile app designed to scan and interpret food labels, making it easier to identify inflammatory ingredients.

Blended Beverages

Berry Turmeric Twist

Servings: 2

Preparation time: 5 minutes

Cooking time: 0 minutes

Ingredients:

- 1 cup mixed berries (fresh or frozen)
- 1 banana
- 1/2 teaspoon ground turmeric
- 1 tablespoon chia seeds
- 1 cup almond milk
- 1 teaspoon honey (optional)
- A pinch of black pepper (to enhance turmeric absorption)
- Ice cubes (optional)

Directions:

1. Place all ingredients in a blender.

2. Blend on high until smooth and creamy.

3. Taste and adjust sweetness with honey if desired.

4. Serve immediately, garnished with a few whole berries on top if desired.

Per serving: Calories: 150, Carbs: 28g, Fiber: 6g, Sugars: 15g, Protein: 3g, Saturated fat: 0.5g, Unsaturated fat: 2g

Difficulty rating: ★☆☆☆

Green Ginger Glow

Servings: 2

Preparation time: 5 minutes

Cooking time: 0 minutes

Ingredients:

- 2 cups spinach leaves
- 1/2 cucumber, chopped
- 1 apple, cored and sliced
- 1 tablespoon fresh ginger, grated
- Juice of 1 lemon
- 1 cup coconut water
- 1 tablespoon flaxseeds
- Ice cubes (optional)

Directions:

1. Combine spinach, cucumber, apple, ginger, lemon juice, and coconut water in a blender.

2. Add flaxseeds and ice cubes if using.

3. Blend until smooth and vibrant green.

4. Pour into glasses and serve immediately for maximum freshness.

Per serving: Calories: 120, Carbs: 25g, Fiber: 5g, Sugars: 14g, Protein: 3g, Saturated fat: 0g, Unsaturated fat: 1g

Difficulty rating: ★☆☆☆

Spicy Pineapple Detox

Servings: 2

Preparation time: 5 minutes

Cooking time: 0 minutes

Ingredients:

- 2 cups pineapple chunks
- 1/2 teaspoon cayenne pepper
- 1 tablespoon apple cider vinegar
- 1 cup water or coconut water
- Juice of 1 lime
- 1 teaspoon honey (optional)
- Mint leaves for garnish (optional)
- Ice cubes (optional)

Directions:

1. Place pineapple, cayenne pepper, apple cider vinegar, water/coconut water, lime juice, and honey (if using) in a blender.

2. Blend until smooth. Adjust sweetness with more honey if needed.

3. Pour into glasses over ice if desired and garnish with mint leaves.

4. Serve immediately, stirring well before drinking.

Per serving: Calories: 100, Carbs: 25g, Fiber: 2g, Sugars: 20g, Protein: 1g, Saturated fat: 0g, Unsaturated fat: 0g

Difficulty rating: ★★☆☆☆

Kale and Apple Morning Shake

Servings: 2

Preparation time: 5 minutes

Cooking time: 0 minutes

Ingredients:

- 1 cup kale, stems removed
- 1 large apple, cored and chopped
- 1 banana
- ½ cup unsweetened almond milk
- ½ cup Greek yogurt
- 1 tablespoon chia seeds
- 1 teaspoon honey (optional)
- Ice cubes (optional)

Directions:

1. Place kale, apple, banana, almond milk, Greek yogurt, chia seeds, and honey (if using) in a blender.

2. Blend on high until smooth. Add ice cubes if a colder shake is desired and blend again.

3. Pour into glasses and serve immediately.

Per serving: Calories: 190, Carbs: 35g, Fiber: 6g, Sugars: 22g, Protein: 8g, Saturated fat: 0.5g, Unsaturated fat: 2g

Difficulty rating: ★☆☆☆☆

Beetroot and Berry Liver Cleanse

Servings: 2

Preparation time: 10 minutes

Cooking time: 0 minutes

Ingredients:

- 1 medium beetroot, peeled and chopped
- 1 cup mixed berries (fresh or frozen)
- 1 small apple, cored and chopped
- ½ lemon, juiced
- 1 tablespoon flaxseed
- 1 cup water
- 1 teaspoon honey (optional)

Directions:

1. Combine beetroot, mixed berries, apple, lemon juice, flaxseed, and water in a blender.

2. Blend on high until completely smooth. Add honey if a sweeter taste is desired and blend again.

3. Strain through a fine mesh sieve if a smoother texture is preferred. Serve immediately.

Per serving: Calories: 145, Carbs: 34g, Fiber: 8g, Sugars: 24g, Protein: 3g, Saturated fat: 0g, Unsaturated fat: 1g

Difficulty rating: ★★☆☆☆

Carrot Ginger Immunity Booster

Servings: 2

Preparation time: 10 minutes

Cooking time: 0 minutes

Ingredients:

- 4 large carrots, washed and peeled
- 1 inch fresh ginger root, peeled
- 1 medium orange, peeled and seeds removed
- 1 tablespoon lemon juice
- 1 teaspoon turmeric powder
- 1 cup water or coconut water
- A pinch of black pepper
- Ice cubes (optional)

Directions:

1. Cut the carrots and ginger root into small pieces suitable for your blender.

2. Place the carrots, ginger, and orange pieces into the blender.

3. Add lemon juice, turmeric powder, and a pinch of black pepper.

4. Pour in 1 cup of water or coconut water for a smoother consistency.

5. Blend on high until smooth. If the mixture is too thick, you can add more water to reach your desired consistency.

6. Serve immediately over ice cubes if preferred.

Per serving: Calories: 95, Carbs: 22g, Fiber: 6g, Sugars: 12g, Protein: 2g, Saturated fat: 0g, Unsaturated fat: 0g

Difficulty rating: ★☆☆☆☆

Citrus Ginger Flush

Servings: 2

Preparation time: 5 minutes

Cooking time: 0 minutes

Ingredients:

- 1 grapefruit, peeled and segmented
- 1 orange, peeled and segmented
- 1/2 lemon, juiced
- 1-inch piece of fresh ginger, peeled
- 1 teaspoon honey (optional)
- 1 cup ice cubes
- A pinch of cayenne pepper (to boost metabolism and enhance absorption of nutrients)

Directions:

1. Place grapefruit, orange, lemon juice, and ginger in a blender.

2. Add honey if a sweeter taste is desired.

3. Include ice cubes for a chilled beverage.

4. Sprinkle in a pinch of cayenne pepper.

5. Blend on high until smooth.

6. Serve immediately, enjoying the vibrant, invigorating flavors that also help reduce inflammation.

Per serving: Calories: 120, Carbs: 30g, Fiber: 3g, Sugars: 20g, Protein: 2g, Saturated fat: 0g, Unsaturated fat: 0g

Difficulty rating: ★☆☆☆☆

Cucumber Mint Refresh

Servings: 2

Preparation time: 5 minutes

Cooking time: 0 minutes

Ingredients:

- 1 large cucumber, chopped
- 1 tablespoon fresh mint leaves
- 2 tablespoons lime juice
- 1 teaspoon grated ginger
- 1 cup cold water
- Ice cubes
- 1 teaspoon honey (optional)

Directions:

1. Place cucumber, mint leaves, lime juice, grated ginger, and water in a blender.

2. Blend on high until smooth. Add honey if desired and blend again.

3. Pour over ice cubes in glasses and serve immediately.

Per serving: Calories: 25, Carbs: 6g, Fiber: 1g, Sugars: 3g, Protein: 1g, Saturated fat: 0g, Unsaturated fat: 0g

Difficulty rating: ★☆☆☆☆

Awakening Breakfasts

Almond Butter and Banana Toast

Servings: 2

Preparation Time: 5 minutes

Cooking time: 2 minutes

Ingredients:

- 2 slices of whole-grain bread
- 2 tablespoons almond butter
- 1 banana, sliced
- 1 teaspoon chia seeds
- A drizzle of honey (optional)

Directions:

1. Toast the whole-grain bread slices to your desired crispness.

2. Spread 1 tablespoon of almond butter on each slice of toast.

3. Arrange banana slices over the almond butter.

4. Sprinkle chia seeds on top for a crunch and an extra dose of nutrients.

5. Drizzle with honey for a touch of sweetness, if desired.

6. Serve immediately for a quick, nutritious breakfast.

Per serving: Calories: 280, Carbs: 30g, Fiber: 5g, Sugars: 10g (not including optional honey), Protein: 8g, Saturated fat: 1g, Unsaturated fat: 8g

Difficulty rating: ★☆☆☆☆

Spinach and Feta Omelette

Servings: 1

Preparation Time: 10 minutes

Cooking time: 6 minutes

Ingredients:

- 2 large eggs
- 1/2 cup fresh spinach, chopped
- 1/4 cup feta cheese, crumbled
- 1 tablespoon olive oil
- Salt and pepper to taste

Directions:

1. In a bowl, whisk the eggs with salt and pepper.

2. Heat olive oil in a skillet over medium heat.

3. Add the spinach to the skillet and sauté until just wilted, about 1-2 minutes.

4. Pour the whisked eggs over the spinach. Cook until the edges start to set, about 2 minutes.

5. Sprinkle feta cheese over half of the omelette. Fold the other half over the cheese.

6. Cook for another 2 minutes, or until the cheese is slightly melted and the eggs are cooked to your liking.

7. Serve immediately.

Per serving: Calories: 290, Carbs: 2g, Fiber: 0g, Sugars: 1g, Protein: 19g, Saturated fat: 7g, Unsaturated fat: 15g

Difficulty rating: ★☆☆☆☆

Turmeric Oatmeal with Blueberries

Servings: 2

Preparation Time: 15 minutes

Cooking time: 12 minutes

Ingredients:

- 1 cup rolled oats
- 2 cups almond milk
- 1/2 teaspoon ground turmeric
- 1 cup fresh blueberries
- 1 tablespoon flaxseeds
- 1 tablespoon maple syrup
- 1/4 teaspoon cinnamon
- A pinch of salt

Directions:

1. In a medium saucepan, bring the almond milk to a low boil.

2. Stir in the rolled oats, ground turmeric, cinnamon, and a pinch of salt. Reduce heat to low.

3. Simmer for 10-12 minutes, stirring occasionally, until the oats are soft and have absorbed most of the liquid.

4. Remove from heat and let it sit for 2 minutes to thicken.

5. Serve the oatmeal in bowls topped with fresh blueberries, flaxseeds, and a drizzle of maple syrup for sweetness.

Per serving: Calories: 280, Carbs: 49g, Fiber: 7g, Sugars: 15g, Protein: 6g, Saturated fat: 0.5g, Unsaturated fat: 3g

Difficulty rating: ★☆☆☆☆

Avocado and Egg Breakfast Bowl

Servings: 2

Preparation Time: 15 minutes

Cooking time: 10 minutes

Ingredients:

- 2 eggs
- 1 avocado, halved and pitted
- 1 cup quinoa, cooked
- 1/2 cup cherry tomatoes, halved
- 1 tablespoon olive oil
- Salt and pepper to taste
- A sprinkle of paprika

Directions:

1. Cook the eggs to your preference (boiled, poached, or scrambled).

2. In two bowls, evenly distribute the cooked quinoa as the base.

3. Place half an avocado in each bowl, sliced or mashed.

4. Add the cooked eggs next to the avocado.

5. Scatter cherry tomatoes around the bowls.

6. Drizzle olive oil over each bowl and season with salt, pepper, and a sprinkle of paprika.

7. Serve immediately for a fulfilling and balanced breakfast.

Per serving: Calories: 400, Carbs: 30g, Fiber: 8g, Sugars: 4g, Protein: 12g, Saturated fat: 3g, Unsaturated fat: 12g

Difficulty rating: ★★☆☆☆

Ginger Pear Smoothie Bowl

Servings: 2

Preparation Time: 10 minutes

Cooking time: 0 minutes

Ingredients:

- 2 ripe pears, cored and chopped
- 1 banana, sliced
- 1/2 teaspoon fresh ginger, grated
- 1 cup spinach leaves
- 1/2 cup almond milk
- Toppings: sliced almonds, chia seeds, and additional pear slices

Directions:

1. In a blender, combine the pears, banana, fresh ginger, spinach leaves, and almond milk. Blend until smooth.

2. Pour the smoothie mixture into bowls.

3. Garnish with sliced almonds, chia seeds, and pear slices for added texture and nutrients.

4. Enjoy this refreshing and energizing smoothie bowl as a vibrant start to your day.

Per serving: Calories: 210, Carbs: 45g, Fiber: 8g, Sugars: 30g, Protein: 3g, Saturated fat: 0g, Unsaturated fat: 2g

Difficulty rating: ★☆☆☆☆

Quinoa Breakfast Bowl with Avocado

Servings: 2

Preparation time: 5 minutes

Cooking time: 15 minutes

Ingredients:

- 1 cup cooked quinoa
- 1 ripe avocado, sliced
- 2 eggs, poached or soft-boiled
- 1 cup spinach leaves, raw or slightly wilted
- 1 tablespoon olive oil
- Salt and pepper to taste
- Toppings: Pumpkin seeds and a squeeze of lemon juice

Directions:

1. Divide the cooked quinoa between two bowls.

2. Top each bowl with half of the sliced avocado and one egg.

3. Arrange spinach leaves around the sides of the bowl.

4. Drizzle olive oil over each bowl and season with salt and pepper.

5. Garnish with pumpkin seeds and a squeeze of lemon juice before serving.

6. Serve immediately for best flavor.

Per serving: Calories: 360, Carbs: 30g, Fiber: 8g, Sugars: 2g, Protein: 12g, Saturated fat: 3g, Unsaturated fat: 10g

Difficulty rating: ★★★☆☆

Chia Seed Pudding with Mixed Berries

Servings: 2

Preparation time: 10 minutes (plus overnight soaking)

Cooking time: 0 minutes

Ingredients:

- 1/4 cup chia seeds
- 1 cup unsweetened almond milk
- 1/2 teaspoon vanilla extract
- 1 tablespoon maple syrup or honey (optional)
- 1 cup mixed berries (fresh or frozen)
- A pinch of salt

Directions:

1. In a bowl, mix chia seeds, almond milk, vanilla extract, sweetener (if using), and a pinch of salt.

2. Stir well until the mixture begins to thicken.

3. Cover and refrigerate overnight, or at least 6 hours.

4. Before serving, stir the pudding to break up any clumps.

5. Serve topped with mixed berries.

Per serving: Calories: 180, Carbs: 24g, Fiber: 10g, Sugars: 8g (varies if sweetener is added), Protein: 5g, Saturated fat: 0.5g, Unsaturated fat: 3g

Difficulty rating: ★☆☆☆☆

Turmeric Oatmeal with Almonds

Servings: 2

Preparation time: 5 minutes

Cooking time: 10 minutes

Ingredients:

- 1 cup rolled oats
- 2 cups water or milk of choice
- 1/2 teaspoon ground turmeric
- 1/4 teaspoon ground cinnamon
- 1 tablespoon maple syrup or honey (optional)
- 1/4 cup almonds, chopped
- A pinch of salt

Directions:

1. In a medium saucepan, bring water or milk to a boil.

2. Add oats, turmeric, cinnamon, and a pinch of salt to the boiling liquid.

3. Reduce heat to low and simmer, stirring occasionally, until oats are soft, about 10 minutes.

4. Remove from heat and let sit for 2 minutes.

5. Stir in maple syrup or honey if using.

6. Serve topped with chopped almonds.

Per serving: Calories: 235, Carbs: 38g, Fiber: 6g, Sugars: 5g (varies if sweetener is added), Protein: 8g, Saturated fat: 0.5g, Unsaturated fat: 4g

Difficulty rating: ★★☆☆☆

Spinach and Feta Omelette

Servings: 1

Preparation time: 5 minutes

Cooking time: 5 minutes

Ingredients:

- 2 large eggs
- 1 tablespoon water
- 1/4 teaspoon black pepper
- 1/4 cup fresh spinach, chopped
- 1/4 cup feta cheese, crumbled
- 1 teaspoon olive oil

Directions:

1. In a bowl, whisk together eggs, water, and black pepper until well combined.

2. Heat olive oil in a non-stick skillet over medium heat.

3. Add spinach to the skillet and sauté until just wilted, about 1 minute.

4. Pour the egg mixture over the spinach. Cook until the edges start to set, about 2 minutes.

5. Sprinkle feta cheese over half of the omelette. Fold the other half over the cheese.

6. Continue to cook until the cheese is melted and the eggs are set, about 2 more minutes.

7. Carefully slide the omelette onto a plate and serve immediately.

Per serving: Calories: 250, Carbs: 2g, Fiber: 0g, Sugars: 1g, Protein: 16g, Saturated fat: 6g, Unsaturated fat: 5g

Difficulty rating: ★★☆☆

Ginger Pear Smoothie Bowl

Servings: 2

Preparation time: 10 minutes

Cooking time: 0 minutes

Ingredients:

- 2 ripe pears, cored and sliced
- 1 banana, peeled
- 1 tablespoon fresh ginger, grated
- 1/2 cup unsweetened almond milk
- 1/2 cup Greek yogurt, plain
- 1 tablespoon chia seeds
- Toppings: Sliced almonds, fresh berries, and a drizzle of honey (optional)

Directions:

1. Place pears, banana, ginger, almond milk, and Greek yogurt in a blender.

2. Blend on high until smooth.

3. Stir in chia seeds and let the mixture sit for 5 minutes to thicken slightly.

4. Pour the smoothie mixture into bowls.

5. Garnish with sliced almonds, fresh berries, and a drizzle of honey if desired.

6. Serve immediately.

Per serving: Calories: 220, Carbs: 42g, Fiber: 7g, Sugars: 28g, Protein: 8g, Saturated fat: 0.5g, Unsaturated fat: 2g

Difficulty rating: ★★☆☆

Pumpkin Spice Oatmeal

Servings: 2

Preparation time: 5 minutes

Cooking time: 15 minutes

Ingredients:

- 1 cup rolled oats
- 1 ¾ cups almond milk
- ½ cup pumpkin puree
- 1 teaspoon pumpkin pie spice
- ¼ teaspoon salt
- 2 tablespoons maple syrup
- ¼ cup chopped almonds
- Additional almond milk for serving (optional)

Directions:

1. In a medium saucepan, bring the almond milk to a boil over medium heat.

2. Add the rolled oats and salt, stirring occasionally, until the oats begin to soften, about 5 minutes.

3. Stir in the pumpkin puree, pumpkin pie spice, and maple syrup. Reduce heat to low and cook for another 10 minutes, stirring occasionally, until the mixture is thick and creamy.

4. Serve the oatmeal in bowls, topped with chopped almonds. Add additional almond milk if desired.

Per serving: Calories: 315, Carbs: 45g, Fiber: 8g, Sugars: 12g, Protein: 9g, Saturated fat: 0.5g, Unsaturated fat: 4g

Difficulty rating: ★★☆☆☆

Sweet Potato and Kale Hash

Servings: 2

Preparation time: 10 minutes

Cooking time: 20 minutes

Ingredients:

- 2 medium sweet potatoes, peeled and diced
- 2 cups kale, stems removed and chopped
- 1 medium onion, diced
- 2 cloves garlic, minced
- 2 tablespoons olive oil
- 1/2 teaspoon smoked paprika
- Salt and pepper to taste
- 4 eggs (optional, for serving on top)

Directions:

1. Heat olive oil in a large skillet over medium heat.

2. Add diced sweet potatoes and cook for 10 minutes, stirring occasionally, until they start to soften.

3. Add diced onion and minced garlic to the skillet. Cook for another 5 minutes until onions are translucent.

4. Stir in chopped kale, smoked paprika, salt, and pepper. Cook until kale is wilted and sweet potatoes are tender, about 5 more minutes.

5. In a separate pan, fry or poach eggs to your preference (optional).

6. Serve the hash in bowls, topped with an egg if using.

Per serving: (without egg): Calories: 280, Carbs: 38g, Fiber: 6g, Sugars: 9g, Protein: 5g, Saturated fat: 2g, Unsaturated fat: 10g

Difficulty rating: ★★★☆☆

Berry Almond Overnight Oats

Servings: 2

Preparation time: 8 hours (overnight soaking)

Cooking time: 0 minutes

Ingredients:

- 1 cup rolled oats
- 1 cup unsweetened almond milk
- 1/2 cup mixed berries (fresh or frozen)
- 2 tablespoons chia seeds
- 2 tablespoons sliced almonds
- 1 tablespoon maple syrup or honey (optional)
- 1/2 teaspoon vanilla extract
- A pinch of salt

Directions:

1. In a medium bowl or jar, combine the rolled oats, almond milk, chia seeds, maple syrup or honey (if using), vanilla extract, and a pinch of salt. Stir well to mix.

2. Gently fold in the mixed berries and sliced almonds.

3. Cover and refrigerate overnight, or for at least 8 hours.

4. Before serving, stir the oats well. If the mixture is too thick, add a little more almond milk to reach your desired consistency.

5. Serve cold, topped with additional berries and almonds if desired.

Per serving: Calories: 320, Carbs: 45g, Fiber: 9g, Sugars: 12g, Protein: 10g, Saturated fat: 0.5g, Unsaturated fat: 4g

Difficulty rating: ★☆☆☆

Coconut Yogurt Parfait with Granola

Servings: 2

Preparation time: 10 minutes

Cooking time: 0 minutes

Ingredients:

- 1 cup coconut yogurt
- 1/2 cup granola
- 1/2 cup mixed berries (such as strawberries, blueberries, and raspberries)
- 2 tablespoons shredded coconut
- 1 tablespoon honey or maple syrup (optional)
- A few mint leaves for garnish (optional)

Directions:

1. In two glasses or parfait jars, layer 1/4 cup of coconut yogurt at the bottom.

2. Add a layer of 2 tablespoons of granola over the yogurt.

3. Add a layer of mixed berries on top of the granola.

4. Repeat the layers, starting with the coconut yogurt and ending with a final layer of berries.

5. Drizzle with honey or maple syrup if desired, and sprinkle shredded coconut on top.

6. Garnish with mint leaves for a refreshing touch.

7. Serve immediately or refrigerate until ready to serve.

Per serving: Calories: 280, Carbs: 38g, Fiber: 5g, Sugars: 18g, Protein: 6g, Saturated fat: 4g, Unsaturated fat: 2g

Difficulty rating: ★☆☆☆☆

Vegan Banana Pancakes

Servings: 2 (about 6 pancakes)

Preparation time: 10 minutes

Cooking time: 15 minutes

Ingredients:

- 1 large ripe banana, mashed
- 1 cup all-purpose flour (or gluten-free flour blend)
- 1 tablespoon baking powder
- 1 tablespoon maple syrup, plus more for serving
- 1 cup almond milk
- 1 teaspoon vanilla extract
- 1/4 teaspoon salt
- Coconut oil, for cooking
- Fresh berries and sliced bananas, for serving

Directions:

1. In a large bowl, whisk together the mashed banana, flour, baking powder, maple syrup, almond milk, vanilla extract, and salt until well combined. The batter should be slightly lumpy.

2. Heat a non-stick skillet or griddle over medium heat and brush with a small amount of coconut oil.

3. Pour 1/4 cup of batter onto the skillet for each pancake. Cook until bubbles form on the surface, then flip and cook until golden brown on the other side, about 2-3 minutes per side.

4. Repeat with the remaining batter, adding more coconut oil to the skillet as needed.

5. Serve the pancakes warm, topped with fresh berries, sliced bananas, and a drizzle of maple syrup.

Per serving: Calories: 345, Carbs: 72g, Fiber: 5g, Sugars: 15g, Protein: 8g, Saturated fat: 1g, Unsaturated fat: 2g

Difficulty rating: ★★☆☆☆

Egg Muffins with Spinach and Mushrooms

Servings: 6

Preparation time: 10 minutes

Cooking time: 20 minutes

Ingredients:

- 6 large eggs
- 1 cup fresh spinach, chopped
- 1/2 cup mushrooms, diced
- 1/4 cup onions, finely chopped
- 1/4 cup bell peppers, diced (optional)
- Salt and pepper to taste
- 1/2 teaspoon garlic powder
- Non-stick cooking spray

Directions:

1. Preheat the oven to 375°F (190°C). Spray a muffin tin with non-stick cooking spray.

2. In a large bowl, whisk the eggs until well beaten.

3. Stir in the spinach, mushrooms, onions, bell peppers (if using), salt, pepper, and garlic powder until well combined.

4. Pour the egg mixture evenly into the muffin tin, filling each cup about 2/3 full.

5. Bake in the preheated oven for 20 minutes, or until the egg muffins are set and lightly golden on top.

6. Allow to cool for a few minutes before removing from the muffin tin. Serve warm.

Per serving: Calories: 100, Carbs: 2g, Fiber: 0.5g, Sugars: 1g, Protein: 8g, Saturated fat: 2g, Unsaturated fat: 3g

Difficulty rating: ★★☆☆☆

Almond Butter Toast with Banana

Servings: 1

Preparation time: 5 minutes

Cooking time: 2 minutes

Ingredients:

- 1 slice whole-grain bread
- 2 tablespoons almond butter
- 1 banana, sliced
- A sprinkle of cinnamon (optional)
- A drizzle of honey (optional)

Directions:

1. Toast the whole-grain bread to your liking.

2. Spread the almond butter evenly over the toasted bread.

3. Arrange the banana slices on top of the almond butter.

4. If desired, sprinkle with cinnamon and drizzle with honey for added flavor.

5. Serve immediately.

Per serving: Calories: 330, Carbs: 44g, Fiber: 7g, Sugars: 21g, Protein: 10g, Saturated fat: 1g, Unsaturated fat: 8g

Difficulty rating: ★☆☆☆☆

Savory Quinoa Porridge with Avocado

Servings: 2

Preparation time: 5 minutes

Cooking time: 15 minutes

Ingredients:

- 1 cup quinoa, rinsed
- 2 cups vegetable broth
- 1/2 teaspoon salt
- 1/4 teaspoon black pepper
- 1 avocado, sliced
- 1/4 cup cherry tomatoes, halved
- 2 tablespoons chopped fresh cilantro
- 1 lime, cut into wedges
- 2 tablespoons pumpkin seeds (optional)

Directions:

1. In a medium saucepan, combine quinoa and vegetable broth. Bring to a boil over high heat.

2. Reduce heat to low, cover, and simmer for 15 minutes, or until quinoa is cooked and liquid is absorbed.

3. Season the cooked quinoa with salt and pepper.

4. Divide the quinoa porridge between two bowls. Top each bowl with avocado slices, cherry tomatoes, and fresh cilantro.

5. Squeeze lime wedges over the bowls for added zest. Sprinkle with pumpkin seeds if desired.

6. Serve warm for a comforting and nutritious meal.

Per serving: Calories: 360, Carbs: 50g, Fiber: 10g, Sugars: 3g, Protein: 12g, Saturated fat: 2g, Unsaturated fat: 10g

Difficulty rating: ★★☆☆☆

Quinoa and Berry Breakfast Cups

Servings: 4

Preparation Time: 20 minutes

Cooking time: 15 minutes

Ingredients:

- 2 cups cooked quinoa, cooled
- 1/2 cup mixed berries (blueberries, raspberries, strawberries)
- 1/4 cup nuts (walnuts or almonds), chopped
- 2 tablespoons honey or maple syrup
- 1/2 teaspoon vanilla extract
- 1/4 cup coconut flakes
- 1 cup Greek yogurt or plant-based yogurt

Directions:

1. Preheat the oven to 350°F (175°C).

2. In a bowl, mix the cooked quinoa with honey (or maple syrup) and vanilla extract.

3. Press the quinoa mixture into the bottoms and up the sides of greased muffin tins, forming cups.

4. Bake for 15 minutes, or until the edges are golden brown. Allow to cool.

5. Once cooled, fill each quinoa cup with Greek yogurt or plant-based yogurt.

6. Top with mixed berries, chopped nuts, and coconut flakes.

7. Serve these delightful breakfast cups for a nutritious and satisfying morning treat.

Per serving: Calories: 280, Carbs: 38g, Fiber: 5g, Sugars: 12g, Protein: 10g, Saturated fat: 2g, Unsaturated fat: 5g

Difficulty rating: ★★☆☆☆

Zucchini Bread with Walnuts

Servings: 12

Preparation time: 15 minutes

Cooking time: 50 minutes

Ingredients:

- 2 cups whole wheat flour
- 1 teaspoon baking soda
- ½ teaspoon baking powder
- 1 teaspoon cinnamon
- ½ teaspoon nutmeg
- ¼ teaspoon salt
- 1 cup grated zucchini, excess water squeezed out
- ½ cup unsweetened applesauce
- ¼ cup olive oil
- ½ cup maple syrup
- 2 eggs
- 1 teaspoon vanilla extract
- ½ cup chopped walnuts

Directions:

1. Preheat oven to 350°F (175°C) and grease a 9x5 inch loaf pan.

2. In a large bowl, combine whole wheat flour, baking soda, baking powder, cinnamon, nutmeg, and salt.

3. In another bowl, mix zucchini, applesauce, olive oil, maple syrup, eggs, and vanilla.

4. Combine wet and dry ingredients until just mixed. Fold in walnuts.

5. Pour batter into the loaf pan, smooth the top, and bake for 50 minutes or until a toothpick comes out clean.

6. Cool in pan for 10 minutes, then on a wire rack before slicing.

Per serving: Calories: 210, Carbs: 30g, Fiber: 4g, Sugars: 12g, Protein: 5g, Saturated fat: 1g, Unsaturated fat: 3g

Difficulty rating: ★★★☆☆

Wholesome Snacks

Almond and Cherry Trail Mix

Servings: 4

Preparation Time: 5 minutes

Cooking time: 0 minutes

Ingredients:

- 1 cup raw almonds
- 1/2 cup dried cherries, unsweetened
- 1/2 cup pumpkin seeds
- 1/4 cup sunflower seeds
- 1/2 teaspoon ground cinnamon
- A pinch of sea salt
- 1/4 teaspoon ground turmeric
- 1/4 cup unsweetened coconut flakes

Directions:

1. In a large bowl, combine raw almonds, dried cherries, pumpkin seeds, and sunflower seeds.

2. Sprinkle the mixture with ground cinnamon, a pinch of sea salt, and ground turmeric. Toss well to ensure even coating.

3. Add unsweetened coconut flakes to the mix and toss again.

4. Store the trail mix in an airtight container and keep it handy for a quick, energizing snack.

Per serving: Calories: 300, Carbs: 20g, Fiber: 5g, Sugars: 8g, Protein: 10g, Saturated fat: 2g, Unsaturated fat: 12g

Difficulty rating: ★☆☆☆☆

Carrot Sticks with Almond Butter Dip

Servings: 4

Preparation Time: 5 minutes

Cooking time: 0 minutes

Ingredients:

- 4 large carrots, peeled and cut into sticks
- 1/2 cup almond butter
- 1 tablespoon maple syrup
- 1/2 teaspoon cinnamon
- A pinch of salt

Directions:

1. In a small bowl, mix almond butter, maple syrup, cinnamon, and a pinch of salt until well combined.

2. Arrange carrot sticks on a plate.

3. Serve the almond butter dip alongside the carrot sticks for a sweet and crunchy snack.

Per serving: Calories: 220, Carbs: 18g, Fiber: 4g, Sugars: 10g, Protein: 5g, Saturated fat: 1g, Unsaturated fat: 8g

Difficulty rating: ★☆☆☆☆

Kale Chips with Nutritional Yeast

Servings: 4

Preparation Time: 20 minutes

Cooking time: 15-20 minutes

Ingredients:

- 1 bunch kale, stems removed and leaves torn into bite-sized pieces
- 1 tablespoon olive oil
- 2 tablespoons nutritional yeast
- Salt to taste

Directions:

1. Preheat the oven to 300°F (150°C).

2. In a large bowl, toss kale pieces with olive oil and salt until evenly coated.

3. Arrange kale in a single layer on a baking sheet.

4. Sprinkle nutritional yeast over the kale.

5. Bake for 15-20 minutes, or until crispy.

6. Let cool before serving. Enjoy a nutritious, crunchy snack.

Per serving: Calories: 80, Carbs: 8g, Fiber: 2g, Sugars: 0g, Protein: 4g, Saturated fat: 0.5g, Unsaturated fat: 3.5g

Difficulty rating: ★☆☆☆☆

Mixed Berry Energy Bites

Servings: 8

Preparation Time: 15 minutes

Chilling time: 1 hour

Ingredients:

- 1 cup mixed berries (fresh or frozen and thawed)
- 1 cup oats
- 1/2 cup almond butter
- 1/4 cup honey or maple syrup
- 1/2 cup ground flaxseed
- 1 teaspoon vanilla extract

Directions:

1. In a food processor, blend mixed berries until smooth.

2. In a large bowl, combine berry puree, oats, almond butter, honey (or maple syrup), ground flaxseed, and vanilla extract. Mix until well combined.

3. Roll the mixture into small balls, about 1 inch in diameter.

4. Place the energy bites on a baking sheet lined with parchment paper and refrigerate for at least 1 hour to set.

5. Store in an airtight container in the refrigerator for a quick, energizing snack.

Per serving: Calories: 220, Carbs: 23g, Fiber: 4g, Sugars: 10g, Protein: 6g, Saturated fat: 1g, Unsaturated fat: 9g

Difficulty rating: ★★☆☆☆

Spicy Roasted Chickpeas

Servings: 4

Preparation Time: 25 minutes

Cooking time: 20-25 minutes

Ingredients:

- 2 cups chickpeas, drained and rinsed
- 1 tablespoon olive oil
- 1/2 teaspoon smoked paprika
- 1/4 teaspoon cayenne pepper
- 1/2 teaspoon garlic powder
- Salt to taste

Directions:

1. Preheat the oven to 400°F (200°C).

2. Pat the chickpeas dry with a kitchen towel.

3. In a bowl, toss the chickpeas with olive oil, smoked paprika, cayenne pepper, garlic powder, and salt.

4. Spread the chickpeas on a baking sheet in a single layer.

5. Roast for 20-25 minutes, or until crispy, stirring halfway through.

6. Let cool before serving. Enjoy as a crunchy, spicy snack.

Per serving: Calories: 220, Carbs: 30g, Fiber: 8g, Sugars: 5g, Protein: 10g, Saturated fat: 1g, Unsaturated fat: 7g

Difficulty rating: ★☆☆☆

Avocado Lime Hummus

Servings: 4

Preparation Time: 10 minutes

Cooking time: 0 minutes

Ingredients:

- 1 ripe avocado
- 1 can (15 oz) chickpeas, drained and rinsed
- 2 tablespoons tahini
- Juice of 1 lime
- 1 clove garlic, minced
- Salt to taste
- 1/4 teaspoon cumin
- 2 tablespoons olive oil

Directions:

1. In a food processor, combine the avocado, chickpeas, tahini, lime juice, minced garlic, salt, and cumin.

2. Process until smooth, gradually adding olive oil until you reach a creamy consistency.

3. Adjust seasoning to taste. Serve with vegetable sticks or whole-grain crackers.

Per serving: Calories: 260, Carbs: 20g, Fiber: 7g, Sugars: 2g, Protein: 6g, Saturated fat: 2g, Unsaturated fat: 10g

Difficulty rating: ★☆☆☆

Pumpkin Spice Granola

Servings: 6

Preparation time: 10 minutes

Cooking time: 30 minutes

Ingredients:

- 3 cups rolled oats
- 1 cup pumpkin seeds
- 1/2 cup chopped pecans
- 1/4 cup maple syrup
- 1/4 cup pumpkin puree
- 2 tablespoons coconut oil, melted
- 1 teaspoon vanilla extract
- 2 teaspoons pumpkin pie spice
- 1/2 teaspoon salt

Directions:

1. Preheat oven to 300°F (150°C). Line a large baking sheet with parchment paper.

2. In a large bowl, combine rolled oats, pumpkin seeds, and chopped pecans.

3. In a separate bowl, whisk together maple syrup, pumpkin puree, melted coconut oil, vanilla extract, pumpkin pie spice, and salt.

4. Pour the wet ingredients over the dry ingredients and stir until well coated.

5. Spread the granola mixture in an even layer on the prepared baking sheet.

6. Bake for 30 minutes, stirring every 10 minutes, until granola is golden and crisp.

7. Let cool completely on the baking sheet. The granola will further crisp as it cools.

8. Store in an airtight container.

Per serving: Calories: 320, Carbs: 38g, Fiber: 6g, Sugars: 12g, Protein: 10g, Saturated fat: 5g, Unsaturated fat: 9g

Difficulty rating: ★★☆☆☆

Beetroot and Walnut Dip

Servings: 4

Preparation time: 10 minutes

Cooking time: 0 minutes

Ingredients:

- 2 medium beetroots, cooked and peeled
- 1/2 cup walnuts, toasted
- 2 cloves garlic
- 2 tablespoons lemon juice
- 1/4 cup olive oil
- Salt and pepper to taste
- 1 tablespoon tahini (optional)

Directions:

1. In a food processor, combine the cooked beetroots, toasted walnuts, garlic, and lemon juice.

2. Pulse until the mixture starts to become smooth.

3. With the processor running, gradually add the olive oil until the mixture is completely smooth.

4. Season with salt and pepper to taste. Add tahini if using and pulse again to mix.

5. Transfer the dip to a serving bowl and chill in the refrigerator for at least 30 minutes before serving.

Per serving: Calories: 210, Carbs: 8g, Fiber: 2g, Sugars: 4g, Protein: 4g, Saturated fat: 2g, Unsaturated fat: 10g

Difficulty rating: ★★☆☆☆

Cinnamon Roasted Almonds

Servings: 4

Preparation time: 5 minutes

Cooking time: 15 minutes

Ingredients:

- 2 cups whole almonds
- 1 tablespoon olive oil
- 2 tablespoons maple syrup
- 1 teaspoon ground cinnamon
- 1/4 teaspoon salt

Directions:

1. Preheat oven to 350°F (175°C). Line a baking sheet with parchment paper.

2. In a bowl, mix together olive oil, maple syrup, ground cinnamon, and salt.

3. Add almonds to the bowl and toss until they are evenly coated.

4. Spread the almonds in a single layer on the prepared baking sheet.

5. Bake for 15 minutes, stirring halfway through, until almonds are fragrant and lightly toasted.

6. Let cool before serving.

Per serving: Calories: 280, Carbs: 14g, Fiber: 6g, Sugars: 6g, Protein: 10g, Saturated fat: 1g, Unsaturated fat: 15g

Difficulty rating: ★☆☆☆

Sweet Potato Toasts with Avocado

Servings: 2

Preparation time: 5 minutes

Cooking time: 15 minutes

Ingredients:

- 1 large sweet potato, sliced lengthwise into 1/4 inch thick slices
- 1 ripe avocado
- Juice of 1/2 a lemon
- Salt and pepper to taste
- 1/4 teaspoon chili flakes (optional)
- 2 tablespoons chopped cilantro

Directions:

1. Toast the sweet potato slices in a toaster or toaster oven on high until tender and slightly crispy, about 2-3 cycles depending on the strength of your toaster.

2. In a bowl, mash the avocado with lemon juice, salt, and pepper.

3. Spread the mashed avocado evenly over the sweet potato slices.

4. Sprinkle with chili flakes (if using) and chopped cilantro.

5. Serve immediately as a nutritious and filling snack or light meal.

Per serving: Calories: 230, Carbs: 27g, Fiber: 7g, Sugars: 5g, Protein: 3g, Saturated fat: 2g, Unsaturated fat: 10g

Difficulty rating: ★☆☆☆

Zucchini Muffins with Flaxseeds

Servings: 12

Preparation time: 15 minutes

Cooking time: 20 minutes

Ingredients:

- 1 1/2 cups whole wheat flour
- 3/4 cup ground flaxseed
- 1/2 cup brown sugar
- 2 teaspoons baking soda
- 1 teaspoon baking powder
- 1 teaspoon cinnamon
- 1/2 teaspoon salt
- 2 cups grated zucchini (about 2 medium zucchinis)
- 3/4 cup unsweetened applesauce
- 2 eggs
- 1 teaspoon vanilla extract
- 1/2 cup chopped walnuts (optional)

Directions:

1. Preheat oven to 350°F (175°C) and prepare a muffin tin with liners or non-stick spray.

2. In a large bowl, combine whole wheat flour, ground flaxseed, brown sugar, baking soda, baking powder, cinnamon, and salt.

3. Mix in grated zucchini.

4. In a separate bowl, whisk applesauce, eggs, and vanilla.

5. Stir wet ingredients into dry until just combined; fold in walnuts if using.

6. Fill muffin cups evenly with batter and bake for 20 minutes, or until a toothpick comes out clean.

7. Cool in the pan for 5 minutes, then transfer to a wire rack.

Per serving: Calories: 180, Carbs: 24g, Fiber: 5g, Sugars: 10g, Protein: 5g, Saturated fat: 0.5g, Unsaturated fat: 3g

Difficulty rating: ★★☆☆☆

Sunflower Seed and Cranberry Bars

Servings: 8

Preparation time: 10 minutes (plus chilling time)

Cooking time: 0 minutes

Chilling time: 2 hours

Ingredients:

- 1 cup sunflower seeds
- 1/2 cup dried cranberries
- 1/2 cup rolled oats
- 1/4 cup honey
- 1/4 cup almond butter
- 1 teaspoon vanilla extract
- 1/4 teaspoon salt

Directions:

1. Line an 8x8 inch baking pan with parchment paper.

2. In a large bowl, combine sunflower seeds, dried cranberries, and rolled oats.

3. In a small saucepan over low heat, mix honey and almond butter until well combined and smooth. Remove from heat and stir in vanilla extract and salt.

4. Pour the almond butter mixture over the dry ingredients and stir until everything is evenly coated.

5. Transfer the mixture to the prepared baking pan, pressing down firmly to ensure the mixture is compact.

6. Refrigerate for at least 2 hours, or until set.

7. Cut into bars and serve.

Per serving: Calories: 220, Carbs: 24g, Fiber: 3g, Sugars: 14g, Protein: 6g, Saturated fat: 1g, Unsaturated fat: 9g

Difficulty rating: ★★☆☆☆

Comforting Soups & Stews

Chicken and Vegetable Soup

Servings: 4

Preparation Time: 30 minutes

Cooking time: 20 minutes

Ingredients:

- 2 chicken breasts, cooked and shredded
- 1 tablespoon olive oil
- 1 onion, chopped
- 2 carrots, sliced
- 2 stalks celery, sliced
- 4 cups chicken broth
- 1 cup kale, chopped
- Salt and pepper to taste
- 1 teaspoon dried thyme

Directions:

1. In a large pot, heat olive oil over medium heat. Add onion, carrots, and celery, cooking until softened.

2. Add chicken broth, shredded chicken, and thyme. Bring to a simmer.

3. Add kale and cook until wilted, about 5 minutes.

4. Season with salt and pepper to taste.

5. Serve hot for a comforting and nutritious meal.

Per serving: Calories: 210, Carbs: 10g, Fiber: 2g, Sugars: 3g, Protein: 25g, Saturated fat: 1g, Unsaturated fat: 4g

Difficulty rating: ★★☆☆☆

Sweet Potato and Ginger Soup

Servings: 4

Preparation Time: 30 minutes

Cooking time: 20 minutes

Ingredients:

- 2 large sweet potatoes, peeled and cubed
- 1 tablespoon olive oil
- 1 onion, chopped
- 2 cloves garlic, minced
- 1 tablespoon fresh ginger, grated
- 4 cups vegetable broth
- Salt and pepper to taste
- 1 can coconut milk
- Fresh cilantro for garnish

Directions:

1. Heat olive oil in a large pot over medium heat. Add onion, garlic, and ginger, sautéing until onion is translucent.

2. Add sweet potatoes and vegetable broth. Bring to a boil, then reduce heat and simmer until sweet potatoes are tender, about 20 minutes.

3. Use an immersion blender to puree the soup until smooth.

4. Stir in coconut milk and season with salt and pepper. Heat through.

5. Serve garnished with fresh cilantro.

Per serving: Calories: 250, Carbs: 35g, Fiber: 5g, Sugars: 10g, Protein: 4g, Saturated fat: 10g, Unsaturated fat: 5g

Difficulty rating: ★★☆☆☆

Hearty Lentil Stew

Servings: 6

Preparation Time: 45 minutes

Cooking time: 30 minutes

Ingredients:

- 1 cup dried lentils, rinsed
- 2 tablespoons olive oil
- 1 onion, diced
- 2 carrots, diced
- 2 stalks celery, diced
- 2 cloves garlic, minced
- 1 teaspoon ground turmeric
- 1 teaspoon smoked paprika
- 6 cups vegetable broth
- 1 can diced tomatoes
- Salt and pepper to taste
- Fresh parsley for garnish

Directions:

1. In a large pot, heat olive oil over medium heat. Add onion, carrots, celery, and garlic. Cook until vegetables are softened.

2. Stir in turmeric and smoked paprika, cooking for another minute until fragrant.

3. Add lentils, vegetable broth, and diced tomatoes. Bring to a boil, then reduce heat and simmer, covered, until lentils are tender, about 30 minutes.

4. Season with salt and pepper to taste.

5. Serve garnished with fresh parsley.

Per serving: Calories: 180, Carbs: 25g, Fiber: 8g, Sugars: 5g, Protein: 10g, Saturated fat: 1g, Unsaturated fat: 5g

Difficulty rating: ★★☆☆

Beef and Barley Soup

Servings: 6

Preparation Time: 1 hour

Cooking time: 45 minutes

Ingredients:

- 1 pound lean beef stew meat, cut into cubes
- 2 tablespoons olive oil
- 1 onion, chopped
- 2 carrots, diced
- 2 stalks celery, diced
- 3 cloves garlic, minced
- 6 cups beef broth
- 1 cup barley
- 1 teaspoon dried rosemary
- Salt and pepper to taste
- Fresh parsley for garnish

Directions:

1. In a large pot, heat olive oil over medium-high heat. Add beef cubes and brown on all sides.

2. Add onion, carrots, celery, and garlic, cooking until vegetables start to soften.

3. Pour in beef broth and bring to a boil. Add barley and rosemary.

4. Reduce heat to low, cover, and simmer until barley is tender and beef is cooked through, about 45 minutes.

5. Season with salt and pepper to taste.

6. Serve garnished with fresh parsley.

Per serving: Calories: 350, Carbs: 35g, Fiber: 8g, Sugars: 4g, Protein: 25g, Saturated fat: 2g, Unsaturated fat: 5g

Difficulty rating: ★★☆☆☆

Tomato and White Bean Soup

Servings: 4

Preparation Time: 30 minutes

Cooking time: 25 minutes

Ingredients:

- 1 tablespoon olive oil
- 1 onion, diced
- 2 cloves garlic, minced
- 1 can (15 oz) white beans, drained and rinsed
- 1 can (15 oz) diced tomatoes
- 4 cups vegetable broth
- 1 teaspoon dried basil
- Salt and pepper to taste
- Fresh basil for garnish

Directions:

1. Heat olive oil in a pot over medium heat. Add onion and garlic, sautéing until onion is translucent.

2. Add white beans, diced tomatoes, vegetable broth, and dried basil. Bring to a boil, then reduce heat and simmer for 20 minutes.

3. Use an immersion blender to partially puree the soup, leaving some beans and tomatoes whole for texture.

4. Season with salt and pepper.

5. Serve garnished with fresh basil.

Per serving: Calories: 180, Carbs: 30g, Fiber: 8g, Sugars: 5g, Protein: 10g, Saturated fat: 0.5g, Unsaturated fat: 3.5g

Difficulty rating: ★★☆☆☆

Tomato and Turmeric Stew

Servings: 4

Preparation time: 10 minutes

Cooking time: 30 minutes

Ingredients:

- 1 tablespoon olive oil
- 1 large onion, diced
- 2 cloves garlic, minced
- 2 teaspoons ground turmeric
- 1 teaspoon ground cumin
- 1/2 teaspoon red pepper flakes
- 4 cups vegetable broth
- 2 cans (14.5 oz each) diced tomatoes, undrained
- 1 can (15 oz) chickpeas, drained and rinsed
- 2 carrots, peeled and diced
- 1 cup quinoa
- Salt and pepper to taste
- Fresh cilantro, chopped for garnish

Directions:

1. Heat olive oil in a large pot over medium heat. Add onion and garlic, sautéing until softened, about 5 minutes.

2. Stir in turmeric, cumin, and red pepper flakes, cooking for another minute until fragrant.

3. Pour in vegetable broth and diced tomatoes with their juice. Bring to a simmer.

4. Add chickpeas, carrots, and quinoa to the pot. Season with salt and pepper.

5. Cover and simmer for about 20 minutes, or until quinoa is cooked and carrots are tender.

6. Adjust seasoning as needed. Serve hot, garnished with fresh cilantro.

Per serving: Calories: 320, Carbs: 55g, Fiber: 10g, Sugars: 8g, Protein: 12g, Saturated fat: 1g, Unsaturated fat: 4g

Difficulty rating: ★★☆☆☆

Beef and Barley Stew with Carrots

Servings: 6

Preparation time: 15 minutes

Cooking time: 1 hour 30 minutes

Ingredients:

- 1 lb beef stew meat, cut into 1-inch pieces
- 3 tablespoons olive oil
- 1 large onion, chopped
- 3 carrots, peeled and sliced
- 2 celery stalks, sliced
- 3 cloves garlic, minced
- 1 cup pearl barley
- 6 cups beef broth
- 1 teaspoon dried thyme
- 1 bay leaf
- Salt and pepper to taste

Directions:

1. Heat 2 tablespoons of olive oil in a large pot over medium-high heat. Add the beef and cook until browned on all sides. Remove the beef from the pot and set aside.

2. In the same pot, add the remaining tablespoon of olive oil, onion, carrots, celery, and garlic. Cook, stirring occasionally, until the vegetables are softened, about 5 minutes.

3. Return the beef to the pot. Add the barley, beef broth, thyme, bay leaf, salt, and pepper. Bring to a boil.

4. Reduce the heat to low, cover, and simmer for 1 hour and 15 minutes, or until the barley and beef are tender.

5. Remove the bay leaf before serving.

Per serving: Calories: 350, Carbs: 40g, Fiber: 8g, Sugars: 4g, Protein: 25g, Saturated fat: 3g, Unsaturated fat: 5g

Difficulty rating: ★★★☆☆

Creamy Butternut Squash Soup

Servings: 4

Preparation time: 20 minutes

Cooking time: 40 minutes

Ingredients:

- 1 large butternut squash, peeled, seeded, and cubed
- 2 tablespoons olive oil
- 1 medium onion, chopped
- 3 cloves garlic, minced
- 4 cups vegetable broth
- 1 teaspoon ground cinnamon
- 1/2 teaspoon ground nutmeg
- 1 cup coconut milk
- Salt and pepper to taste
- Pumpkin seeds for garnish (optional)

Directions:

1. Heat olive oil in a large pot over medium heat. Add onion and garlic, cooking until soft and translucent, about 5 minutes.

2. Add the cubed butternut squash, vegetable broth, cinnamon, and nutmeg. Season with salt and pepper. Bring to a boil, then reduce heat and simmer until squash is tender, about 25-30 minutes.

3. Use an immersion blender to puree the soup until smooth. Stir in the coconut milk and heat through.

4. Taste and adjust seasoning if necessary. Serve hot, garnished with pumpkin seeds if desired.

Per serving: Calories: 250, Carbs: 30g, Fiber: 5g, Sugars: 8g, Protein: 3g, Saturated fat: 7g, Unsaturated fat: 5g

Difficulty rating: ★★☆☆☆

Chicken and Ginger Broth

Servings: 4

Preparation time: 10 minutes

Cooking time: 40 minutes

Ingredients:

- 1 tablespoon olive oil
- 1 lb chicken breast, cut into bite-sized pieces
- 1 large onion, chopped
- 2 carrots, peeled and sliced
- 2 stalks celery, sliced
- 3 cloves garlic, minced
- 2 inches fresh ginger, peeled and grated
- 6 cups chicken broth
- Salt and pepper to taste
- 2 tablespoons fresh parsley, chopped
- Juice of 1 lemon

Directions:

1. Heat olive oil in a large pot over medium-high heat. Add chicken pieces, cooking until browned on all sides. Remove chicken and set aside.

2. In the same pot, add onion, carrots, celery, garlic, and ginger. Sauté until vegetables are softened, about 5 minutes.

3. Return chicken to the pot. Add chicken broth. Season with salt and pepper.

4. Bring to a boil, then reduce heat and simmer for 30 minutes.

5. Stir in fresh parsley and lemon juice just before serving.

6. Serve hot, adjusting seasoning as needed.

Per serving: Calories: 210, Carbs: 10g, Fiber: 2g, Sugars: 4g, Protein: 28g, Saturated fat: 1g, Unsaturated fat: 3g

Difficulty rating: ★★☆☆☆

Lentil and Spinach Soup

Servings: 4

Preparation time: 10 minutes

Cooking time: 25 minutes

Ingredients:

- 1 tablespoon olive oil
- 1 onion, diced
- 2 cloves garlic, minced
- 1 teaspoon ground cumin
- 1/2 teaspoon ground coriander
- 1 cup red lentils, rinsed
- 4 cups vegetable broth
- 2 cups water
- 1 can (14.5 oz) diced tomatoes, undrained
- 3 cups fresh spinach, roughly chopped
- Salt and pepper to taste
- Lemon wedges for serving

Directions:

1. Heat olive oil in a large pot over medium heat. Add onion and garlic, cooking until softened, about 5 minutes.

2. Stir in cumin and coriander, cooking for another minute until fragrant.

3. Add red lentils, vegetable broth, water, and diced tomatoes to the pot. Season with salt and pepper.

4. Bring to a boil, then reduce heat and simmer for 20 minutes, or until lentils are tender.

5. Stir in spinach and cook until wilted, about 2 minutes.

6. Serve hot, with lemon wedges on the side for squeezing over the soup.

Per serving: Calories: 240, Carbs: 38g, Fiber: 16g, Sugars: 6g, Protein: 14g, Saturated fat: 0.5g, Unsaturated fat: 3g

Difficulty rating: ★☆☆☆☆

Vegetable Minestrone

Servings: 6

Preparation time: 15 minutes

Cooking time: 40 minutes

Ingredients:

- 2 tablespoons olive oil
- 1 large onion, diced
- 2 carrots, peeled and diced
- 2 stalks celery, diced
- 3 cloves garlic, minced
- 1 zucchini, diced
- 1 cup green beans, trimmed and cut into 1-inch pieces
- 1 can (14.5 oz) diced tomatoes
- 6 cups vegetable broth
- 1 can (15 oz) kidney beans, drained and rinsed
- 1 cup small pasta, such as ditalini
- 1 teaspoon dried oregano
- 1 teaspoon dried basil
- Salt and pepper to taste
- Grated Parmesan cheese for garnish (optional)

Directions:

1. Heat olive oil in a large pot over medium heat. Sauté onion, carrots, celery, and garlic until softened, about 5 minutes.

2. Add zucchini and green beans, cooking for an additional 5 minutes.

3. Stir in diced tomatoes, vegetable broth, kidney beans, pasta, oregano, and basil. Season with salt and pepper. Bring to a boil.

4. Reduce heat to low and simmer, covered, for 20 minutes, or until the pasta is cooked and vegetables are tender.

5. Serve hot, garnished with grated Parmesan cheese if desired.

Per serving: Calories: 220, Carbs: 38g, Fiber: 8g, Sugars: 6g, Protein: 9g, Saturated fat: 1g, Unsaturated fat: 3g

Difficulty rating: ★★☆☆

Spicy Black Bean Soup

Servings: 4

Preparation time: 10 minutes

Cooking time: 25 minutes

Ingredients:

- 2 cans (15 oz each) black beans, drained and rinsed
- 1 large onion, chopped
- 2 cloves garlic, minced
- 1 tablespoon olive oil
- 2 teaspoons ground cumin
- 1 teaspoon chili powder
- 1/4 teaspoon cayenne pepper
- 4 cups vegetable broth
- Juice of 1 lime
- Salt and pepper to taste
- Fresh cilantro, for garnish
- Avocado slices, for garnish

Directions:

1. Heat olive oil in a large pot over medium heat. Add onion and garlic, sautéing until softened, about 5 minutes.

2. Stir in cumin, chili powder, and cayenne pepper, cooking for another minute until fragrant.

3. Add black beans and vegetable broth. Bring to a boil, then reduce heat and simmer for 15 minutes.

4. Using an immersion blender, blend the soup until smooth with some whole beans left for texture. Alternatively, carefully transfer to a blender in batches.

5. Stir in lime juice and season with salt and pepper to taste.

6. Serve hot, garnished with fresh cilantro and avocado slices.

Per serving: Calories: 220, Carbs: 34g, Fiber: 10g, Sugars: 2g, Protein: 12g, Saturated fat: 1g, Unsaturated fat: 4g

Difficulty rating: ★★☆☆

Mushroom and Thyme Stew

Servings: 4

Preparation time: 15 minutes

Cooking time: 30 minutes

Ingredients:

- 1 lb mixed mushrooms, roughly chopped
- 1 large carrot, diced
- 1 onion, diced
- 2 cloves garlic, minced
- 2 tablespoons olive oil
- 4 cups vegetable broth
- 1 cup pearl barley, rinsed
- 2 teaspoons fresh thyme leaves
- Salt and pepper to taste
- Fresh parsley, for garnish

Directions:

1. In a large pot, heat olive oil over medium heat. Add onion, carrot, and garlic, sautéing until softened, about 5 minutes.

2. Add mushrooms and cook until they start to release their juices, about 8 minutes.

3. Stir in pearl barley, vegetable broth, and thyme leaves. Bring to a boil, then reduce heat, cover, and simmer for 20 minutes, or until barley is tender.

4. Season with salt and pepper to taste.

5. Serve hot, garnished with fresh parsley.

Per serving: Calories: 260, Carbs: 45g, Fiber: 10g, Sugars: 5g, Protein: 8g, Saturated fat: 1g, Unsaturated fat: 5g

Difficulty rating: ★★★☆☆

Carrot and Coriander Soup

Servings: 4

Preparation time: 10 minutes

Cooking time: 20 minutes

Ingredients:

- 1 lb carrots, peeled and diced
- 1 onion, chopped
- 2 cloves garlic, minced
- 1 tablespoon olive oil
- 4 cups vegetable broth
- 2 teaspoons ground coriander
- 1 teaspoon ground cumin
- Salt and pepper to taste
- Fresh coriander (cilantro), for garnish
- A dollop of yogurt, for serving (optional)

Directions:

1. Heat olive oil in a large pot over medium heat. Add onion and garlic, sautéing until softened, about 5 minutes.

2. Add carrots, vegetable broth, ground coriander, and cumin. Bring to a boil, then reduce heat and simmer for 15 minutes, or until carrots are tender.

3. Using an immersion blender, blend the soup until smooth. Alternatively, carefully transfer to a blender in batches and blend until smooth.

4. Season with salt and pepper to taste.

5. Serve hot, garnished with fresh coriander and a dollop of yogurt if desired.

Per serving: Calories: 120, Carbs: 18g, Fiber: 5g, Sugars: 8g, Protein: 2g, Saturated fat: 0.5g, Unsaturated fat: 3g

Difficulty rating: ★☆☆☆☆

Pea and Mint Soup

Servings: 4

Preparation time: 10 minutes

Cooking time: 20 minutes

Ingredients:

- 4 cups fresh or frozen peas
- 4 cups vegetable broth
- 1/2 cup chopped fresh mint
- 1 medium onion, diced
- 2 cloves garlic, minced
- 2 tablespoons olive oil
- Salt and pepper to taste
- 1/4 cup coconut milk (optional, for garnish)

Directions:

1. In a large pot, heat the olive oil over medium heat. Add the diced onion and minced garlic, sautéing until the onion is translucent, about 5 minutes.

2. Add the peas and vegetable broth to the pot. Bring to a boil, then reduce heat and simmer for 10 minutes.

3. Stir in the chopped mint, and continue to simmer for another 5 minutes.

4. Remove from heat. Use an immersion blender to puree the soup until smooth. Alternatively, carefully transfer the soup to a blender and puree in batches.

5. Season with salt and pepper to taste.

6. Serve hot, garnished with a swirl of coconut milk if desired.

Per serving: Calories: 220, Carbs: 30g, Fiber: 9g, Sugars: 12g, Protein: 9g, Saturated fat: 1g, Unsaturated fat: 6g

Difficulty rating: ★★☆☆☆

Broccoli and Almond Soup

Servings: 4

Preparation time: 10 minutes

Cooking time: 20 minutes

Ingredients:

- 2 tablespoons olive oil
- 1 onion, chopped
- 2 cloves garlic, minced
- 4 cups broccoli florets
- 4 cups vegetable broth
- 1/2 cup almonds, toasted and chopped
- Salt and pepper to taste
- 1/4 teaspoon nutmeg
- 1 cup almond milk

Directions:

1. Heat olive oil in a large pot over medium heat. Add onion and garlic, sautéing until soft and translucent, about 5 minutes.

2. Add broccoli florets and cook for another 5 minutes, stirring occasionally.

3. Pour in vegetable broth and bring to a boil. Reduce heat and simmer until broccoli is tender, about 10 minutes.

4. Stir in toasted almonds, reserving a few for garnish. Season with salt, pepper, and nutmeg.

5. Using an immersion blender, puree the soup until smooth. Stir in almond milk and heat through.

6. Serve hot, garnished with reserved almonds.

Per serving: Calories: 220, Carbs: 15g, Fiber: 6g, Sugars: 5g, Protein: 8g, Saturated fat: 1g, Unsaturated fat: 14g

Difficulty rating: ★★☆☆☆

Chicken Noodle Soup with Turmeric

Servings: 6

Preparation time: 15 minutes

Cooking time: 30 minutes

Ingredients:

- 1 lb chicken breast, diced
- 8 cups chicken broth
- 2 cups egg noodles
- 1 cup carrots, diced
- 1 cup celery, diced
- 1 medium onion, diced
- 3 cloves garlic, minced
- 2 teaspoons turmeric
- 1 teaspoon dried thyme
- 2 tablespoons olive oil
- Salt and pepper to taste
- Fresh parsley, chopped (for garnish)

Directions:

1. In a large pot, heat the olive oil over medium heat. Add the diced onion, carrots, celery, and minced garlic. Sauté until the vegetables are softened, about 5 minutes.

2. Add the diced chicken breast to the pot and cook until the chicken is no longer pink on the outside, about 5 minutes.

3. Pour in the chicken broth and bring the mixture to a boil.

4. Once boiling, reduce the heat to a simmer and add the turmeric, dried thyme, salt, and pepper. Stir well to combine.

5. Add the egg noodles to the pot and simmer for 10 minutes, or until the noodles are tender.

6. Taste and adjust seasoning if necessary.

7. Serve hot, garnished with fresh parsley.

Per serving: Calories: 290, Carbs: 22g, Fiber: 2g, Sugars: 3g, Protein: 25g, Saturated fat: 2g, Unsaturated fat: 4g

Difficulty rating: ★★☆☆☆

Cauliflower and Turmeric Chowder

Servings: 4

Preparation time: 15 minutes

Cooking time: 25 minutes

Ingredients:

- 2 tablespoons coconut oil
- 1 large onion, diced
- 2 cloves garlic, minced
- 1 teaspoon ground turmeric
- 1/2 teaspoon ground cumin
- 1 large head cauliflower, chopped into florets
- 4 cups vegetable broth
- 1 cup coconut milk
- Salt and pepper to taste
- 2 tablespoons chopped cilantro for garnish

Directions:

1. In a large pot, heat coconut oil over medium heat. Add onion and garlic, cooking until onion is translucent, about 5 minutes.

2. Stir in turmeric and cumin, cooking for another minute until fragrant.

3. Add cauliflower florets to the pot, stirring to coat with the spices.

4. Pour in vegetable broth and bring to a boil. Reduce heat to low and simmer until cauliflower is tender, about 15 minutes.

5. Stir in coconut milk and season with salt and pepper. Simmer for an additional 5 minutes.

6. Using an immersion blender, blend the chowder until smooth with some chunks of cauliflower remaining for texture.

7. Serve hot, garnished with chopped cilantro.

Per serving: Calories: 210, Carbs: 18g, Fiber: 5g, Sugars: 6g, Protein: 5g, Saturated fat: 14g, Unsaturated fat: 4g

Difficulty rating: ★★☆☆☆

Fresh Salads & Sides

Avocado Quinoa Salad

Servings: 4

Preparation Time: 20 minutes

Cooking time: 0 minutes

Ingredients:

- 2 cups cooked quinoa, cooled
- 1 ripe avocado, diced
- 1/2 cup cucumber, diced
- 1/4 cup red onion, finely chopped
- 1/2 cup cherry tomatoes, halved
- 1/4 cup fresh cilantro, chopped
- 2 tablespoons lime juice
- 2 tablespoons extra-virgin olive oil
- Salt and pepper to taste

Directions:

1. In a large bowl, combine cooled quinoa, diced avocado, cucumber, red onion, cherry tomatoes, and cilantro.

2. In a small bowl, whisk together lime juice, olive oil, salt, and pepper to create the dressing.

3. Drizzle the dressing over the salad and gently toss to combine, ensuring not to mash the avocado pieces.

4. Adjust seasoning if necessary and serve chilled or at room temperature.

Per serving: Calories: 250, Carbs: 25g, Fiber: 6g, Sugars: 3g, Protein: 5g, Saturated fat: 2g, Unsaturated fat: 10g

Difficulty rating: ★☆☆☆☆

Zesty Lemon Broccoli

Servings: 4

Preparation Time: 15 minutes

Cooking time: 5-7 minutes

Ingredients:

- 4 cups broccoli florets
- 2 tablespoons olive oil
- Salt and pepper to taste
- Zest of 1 lemon
- 2 tablespoons lemon juice
- 1/4 cup slivered almonds

Directions:

1. Steam broccoli florets until just tender, about 5-7 minutes.

2. In a large skillet, heat olive oil over medium heat. Add steamed broccoli, salt, and pepper. Sauté for 2-3 minutes.

3. Remove from heat and add lemon zest, lemon juice, and slivered almonds. Toss to combine.

4. Serve immediately, offering a bright and tangy flavor to complement any main dish.

Per serving: Calories: 150, Carbs: 10g, Fiber: 3g, Sugars: 2g, Protein: 4g, Saturated fat: 1g, Unsaturated fat: 9g

Difficulty rating: ★☆☆☆☆

Crunchy Rainbow Salad

Servings: 4

Preparation Time: 15 minutes

Cooking time: 0 minutes

Ingredients:

- 2 cups kale, chopped
- 1 cup red cabbage, shredded
- 1 large carrot, julienned
- 1 bell pepper (red or yellow), thinly sliced
- 1/2 cup cherry tomatoes, halved
- 1/4 cup almonds, sliced
- 2 tablespoons olive oil
- 1 tablespoon apple cider vinegar
- Salt and pepper to taste
- 1 tablespoon hemp seeds

Directions:

1. In a large salad bowl, combine kale, red cabbage, carrot, bell pepper, and cherry tomatoes.

2. In a small bowl, whisk together olive oil, apple cider vinegar, salt, and pepper to create the dressing.

3. Pour the dressing over the salad and toss until all ingredients are well coated.

4. Sprinkle sliced almonds and hemp seeds on top for added crunch and nutrition.

5. Serve immediately or let it sit for 10 minutes to allow the kale to soften slightly.

Per serving: Calories: 150, Carbs: 10g, Fiber: 4g, Sugars: 4g, Protein: 5g, Saturated fat: 1g, Unsaturated fat: 9g

Difficulty rating: ★☆☆☆☆

Cucumber and Dill Salad

Servings: 4

Preparation time: 10 minutes

Cooking time: 0 minutes

Ingredients:

- 2 large cucumbers, thinly sliced
- 1/4 cup red onion, thinly sliced
- 1/4 cup fresh dill, chopped
- 3 tablespoons olive oil
- 2 tablespoons white wine vinegar
- 1 teaspoon sugar
- Salt and pepper to taste

Directions:

1. In a large bowl, combine the thinly sliced cucumbers, red onion, and chopped dill.

2. In a small bowl, whisk together olive oil, white wine vinegar, sugar, salt, and pepper until the sugar is dissolved.

3. Pour the dressing over the cucumber mixture and toss gently to coat.

4. Refrigerate for at least 30 minutes before serving to allow the flavors to blend.

5. Serve chilled as a refreshing side dish.

Per serving: Calories: 120, Carbs: 6g, Fiber: 1g, Sugars: 4g, Protein: 1g, Saturated fat: 1g, Unsaturated fat: 9g

Difficulty rating: ★☆☆☆☆

Roasted Butternut Squash with Pecans

Servings: 4

Preparation Time: 40 minutes

Cooking time: 30 minutes

Ingredients:

- 1 medium butternut squash, peeled, seeded, and cubed
- 2 tablespoons olive oil
- Salt and pepper to taste
- 1/2 cup pecans, roughly chopped
- 2 tablespoons maple syrup
- 1/4 teaspoon ground cinnamon

Directions:

1. Preheat the oven to 400°F (200°C).

2. Toss butternut squash cubes with olive oil, salt, and pepper. Spread on a baking sheet in a single layer.

3. Roast in the oven for 25-30 minutes, or until squash is tender and lightly caramelized, stirring halfway through.

4. In the last 5 minutes of roasting, sprinkle chopped pecans over the squash.

5. Drizzle maple syrup and sprinkle ground cinnamon over the roasted squash and pecans. Toss lightly to coat.

6. Serve warm as a flavorful and nutritious side dish.

Per serving: Calories: 260, Carbs: 30g, Fiber: 5g, Sugars: 12g, Protein: 3g, Saturated fat: 1g, Unsaturated fat: 12g

Difficulty rating: ★★☆☆☆

Quinoa and Black Bean Salad

Servings: 4

Preparation time: 15 minutes

Cooking time: 20 minutes

Ingredients:

- 1 cup quinoa
- 2 cups water
- 1 can (15 oz) black beans, drained and rinsed
- 1 red bell pepper, diced
- 1/4 cup fresh cilantro, chopped
- 1/4 cup lime juice
- 2 tablespoons olive oil
- 1/2 teaspoon ground cumin
- Salt and pepper to taste
- 1 avocado, diced

Directions:

1. Rinse quinoa under cold water until water runs clear.

2. In a medium saucepan, bring 2 cups of water to a boil. Add quinoa, reduce heat to low, cover, and simmer for 15 minutes or until water is absorbed. Remove from heat and let stand for 5 minutes. Fluff with a fork and allow to cool.

3. In a large bowl, combine cooled quinoa, black beans, red bell pepper, and cilantro.

4. In a small bowl, whisk together lime juice, olive oil, ground cumin, salt, and pepper. Pour over the quinoa mixture and toss to coat evenly.

5. Gently fold in diced avocado.

6. Serve chilled or at room temperature.

Per serving: Calories: 320, Carbs: 45g, Fiber: 10g, Sugars: 3g, Protein: 10g, Saturated fat: 2g, Unsaturated fat: 7g

Difficulty rating: ★★☆☆☆

Roasted Beet and Goat Cheese Salad

Servings: 4

Preparation time: 15 minutes

Cooking time: 45 minutes

Ingredients:

- 4 medium beets, peeled and cubed
- 2 tablespoons olive oil
- Salt and pepper to taste
- 6 cups mixed greens (such as arugula and spinach)
- 1/2 cup walnuts, toasted and chopped
- 1/4 cup balsamic vinegar
- 1/2 cup goat cheese, crumbled
- 2 tablespoons honey

Directions:

1. Preheat oven to 400°F (200°C). Toss cubed beets with olive oil, salt, and pepper. Spread on a baking sheet and roast for 45 minutes, or until tender, stirring occasionally. Let cool.

2. In a large bowl, combine mixed greens and cooled roasted beets.

3. In a small skillet over medium heat, toast walnuts until fragrant, about 5 minutes. Let cool, then add to the salad.

4. In a small bowl, whisk together balsamic vinegar and honey. Drizzle over the salad.

5. Top salad with crumbled goat cheese.

6. Serve immediately.

Per serving: Calories: 290, Carbs: 20g, Fiber: 4g, Sugars: 16g, Protein: 8g, Saturated fat: 5g, Unsaturated fat: 10g

Difficulty rating: ★★☆☆☆

Avocado and Spinach Salad with Lemon Dressing

Servings: 4

Preparation time: 10 minutes

Cooking time: 0 minutes

Ingredients:

- 6 cups fresh spinach leaves
- 1 ripe avocado, sliced
- 1/4 cup red onion, thinly sliced
- 1/4 cup almonds, sliced and toasted
- For the dressing:
- 2 tablespoons olive oil
- 2 tablespoons lemon juice
- 1 teaspoon honey
- 1 clove garlic, minced
- Salt and pepper to taste

Directions:

1. In a large salad bowl, combine spinach leaves, sliced avocado, and red onion.

2. In a dry skillet over medium heat, toast sliced almonds until golden and fragrant. Sprinkle over the salad.

3. In a small bowl, whisk together olive oil, lemon juice, honey, minced garlic, salt, and pepper until well combined.

4. Drizzle the dressing over the salad and toss gently to coat.

5. Serve immediately.

Per serving: Calories: 220, Carbs: 14g, Fiber: 6g, Sugars: 4g, Protein: 4g, Saturated fat: 2g, Unsaturated fat: 10g

Difficulty rating: ★☆☆☆☆

Kale and Almond Salad

Servings: 4

Preparation time: 15 minutes

Cooking time: 0 minutes

Ingredients:

- 4 cups kale, stems removed and leaves torn
- 1/2 cup sliced almonds, toasted
- 1/4 cup dried cranberries
- 1/4 cup shaved Parmesan cheese
- 2 tablespoons olive oil
- 1 tablespoon apple cider vinegar
- 1 teaspoon honey
- Salt and pepper to taste

Directions:

1. In a large bowl, combine the kale, toasted almonds, dried cranberries, and shaved Parmesan cheese.

2. In a small bowl, whisk together olive oil, apple cider vinegar, honey, salt, and pepper until well blended.

3. Pour the dressing over the kale mixture and toss to coat evenly.

4. Let the salad sit for about 10 minutes to allow the kale to soften slightly.

5. Serve as a refreshing side dish or a light main course.

Per serving: Calories: 220, Carbs: 14g, Fiber: 3g, Sugars: 7g, Protein: 7g, Saturated fat: 2g, Unsaturated fat: 10g

Difficulty rating: ★☆☆☆☆

Carrot and Apple Slaw

Servings: 4

Preparation time: 20 minutes

Cooking time: 0 minutes

Ingredients:

- 3 large carrots, peeled and grated
- 1 large apple, cored and thinly sliced
- 1/4 cup raisins
- 2 tablespoons mayonnaise
- 1 tablespoon honey
- 1 tablespoon apple cider vinegar
- Salt and pepper to taste
- 2 tablespoons chopped fresh parsley

Directions:

1. In a large bowl, combine grated carrots, thinly sliced apple, and raisins.

2. In a small bowl, whisk together mayonnaise, honey, and apple cider vinegar until smooth. Season with salt and pepper.

3. Pour the dressing over the carrot and apple mixture. Toss to coat evenly.

4. Refrigerate for at least 15 minutes to allow flavors to meld.

5. Just before serving, sprinkle with chopped fresh parsley for added freshness.

Per serving: Calories: 140, Carbs: 24g, Fiber: 3g, Sugars: 18g, Protein: 1g, Saturated fat: 1g, Unsaturated fat: 2g

Difficulty rating: ★☆☆☆☆

Mediterranean Chickpea Salad

Servings: 4

Preparation Time: 15 minutes

Cooking time: 0 minutes

Ingredients:

- 1 can (15 oz) chickpeas, drained and rinsed
- 1 cup English cucumber, diced
- 1 cup cherry tomatoes, halved
- 1/2 cup Kalamata olives, pitted and halved
- 1/4 cup red onion, thinly sliced
- 1/4 cup feta cheese, crumbled (optional for vegan)
- 2 tablespoons extra-virgin olive oil
- 1 tablespoon lemon juice
- 1 teaspoon dried oregano
- Salt and pepper to taste

Directions:

1. In a large bowl, combine chickpeas, cucumber, cherry tomatoes, Kalamata olives, and red onion.

2. If using, sprinkle feta cheese over the salad.

3. In a small bowl, whisk together olive oil, lemon juice, dried oregano, salt, and pepper to create the dressing.

4. Pour the dressing over the salad and toss to ensure all ingredients are evenly coated.

5. Serve immediately or chill in the refrigerator for 30 minutes to allow flavors to meld.

Per serving: Calories: 220, Carbs: 20g, Fiber: 5g, Sugars: 5g, Protein: 7g, Saturated fat: 3g, Unsaturated fat: 10g

Difficulty rating: ★☆☆☆☆

Sweet Potato and Quinoa Salad

Servings: 4

Preparation time: 20 minutes

Cooking time: 30 minutes

Ingredients:

- 2 medium sweet potatoes, peeled and cubed
- 1 cup quinoa, rinsed
- 2 cups water
- 1/4 cup olive oil, divided
- Salt and pepper to taste
- 1/4 cup red onion, finely chopped
- 1/4 cup fresh parsley, chopped
- 1/4 cup dried cranberries
- 1/4 cup toasted, chopped pecans
- 2 tablespoons apple cider vinegar

Directions:

1. Preheat the oven to 400°F (200°C). Toss sweet potatoes with 2 tablespoons of olive oil, salt, and pepper. Spread on a baking sheet and roast for 25-30 minutes, until tender and lightly browned.

2. While sweet potatoes are roasting, bring 2 cups of water to a boil in a medium saucepan. Add quinoa, reduce heat to low, cover, and simmer for 15 minutes, or until water is absorbed. Remove from heat and let sit covered for 5 minutes. Fluff with a fork.

3. In a large bowl, combine roasted sweet potatoes, cooked quinoa, red onion, parsley, dried cranberries, and pecans.

4. In a small bowl, whisk together the remaining 2 tablespoons of olive oil and apple cider vinegar. Pour over the salad and toss to combine. Season with salt and pepper to taste.

5. Serve warm or at room temperature.

Per serving: Calories: 380, Carbs: 50g, Fiber: 7g, Sugars: 9g, Protein: 8g, Saturated fat: 1g, Unsaturated fat: 9g

Difficulty rating: ★★☆☆☆

Broccoli and Cranberry Salad

Servings: 4

Preparation time: 15 minutes

Cooking time: 0 minutes

Ingredients:

- 4 cups broccoli florets, finely chopped
- 1/2 cup red onion, finely chopped
- 1/2 cup dried cranberries
- 1/4 cup sunflower seeds
- 1/4 cup almonds, sliced and toasted
- 1/2 cup Greek yogurt
- 2 tablespoons apple cider vinegar
- 1 tablespoon honey
- Salt and pepper to taste

Directions:

1. In a large bowl, combine broccoli florets, red onion, dried cranberries, sunflower seeds, and almonds.

2. In a small bowl, whisk together Greek yogurt, apple cider vinegar, honey, salt, and pepper until smooth.

3. Pour the dressing over the broccoli mixture and toss to coat evenly.

4. Refrigerate for at least 30 minutes before serving to allow flavors to meld.

5. Serve chilled or at room temperature.

Per serving: Calories: 220, Carbs: 28g, Fiber: 4g, Sugars: 18g, Protein: 7g, Saturated fat: 0.5g, Unsaturated fat: 5g

Difficulty rating: ★☆☆☆☆

Mixed Berry and Spinach Salad

Servings: 4

Preparation time: 15 minutes

Cooking time: 0 minutes

Ingredients:

- 4 cups fresh spinach leaves, washed and dried
- 1 cup mixed berries (strawberries, blueberries, raspberries)
- 1/2 cup walnuts, toasted and chopped
- 1/4 cup feta cheese, crumbled
- 1/4 cup balsamic vinegar
- 1/2 cup olive oil
- 1 tablespoon honey
- Salt and pepper to taste

Directions:

1. In a large salad bowl, combine spinach leaves, mixed berries, toasted walnuts, and crumbled feta cheese.

2. In a small bowl, whisk together balsamic vinegar, olive oil, honey, salt, and pepper until well combined.

3. Drizzle the dressing over the salad and toss gently to coat all the ingredients.

4. Serve immediately for the freshest taste.

Per serving: Calories: 340, Carbs: 18g, Fiber: 3g, Sugars: 12g, Protein: 5g, Saturated fat: 3g, Unsaturated fat: 24g

Difficulty rating: ★☆☆☆

Cauliflower Tabouleh

Servings: 4

Preparation time: 15 minutes

Cooking time: 0 minutes

Ingredients:

- 1 large head cauliflower, riced
- 1 cup parsley, finely chopped
- 1/2 cup mint, finely chopped
- 2 tomatoes, diced
- 1/4 cup onion, finely diced
- 3 tablespoons olive oil
- Juice of 1 lemon
- Salt and pepper to taste

Directions:

1. Place the riced cauliflower in a large mixing bowl.

2. Add the chopped parsley, mint, diced tomatoes, and onion to the bowl with the cauliflower.

3. Drizzle olive oil and lemon juice over the mixture.

4. Season with salt and pepper to taste.

5. Toss all ingredients until well combined.

6. Refrigerate for at least 30 minutes before serving to allow flavors to meld.

Per serving: Calories: 120, Carbs: 14g, Fiber: 5g, Sugars: 6g, Protein: 3g, Saturated fat: 1g, Unsaturated fat: 9g

Difficulty rating: ★☆☆☆☆

Zucchini Noodle Salad

Servings: 4

Preparation time: 20 minutes

Cooking time: 0 minutes

Ingredients:

- 4 medium zucchinis, spiralized
- 1 cup cherry tomatoes, halved
- 1/2 cup corn kernels, fresh or thawed from frozen
- 1/4 cup red onion, finely chopped
- 1 avocado, diced
- 1/4 cup cilantro, chopped
- 1/4 cup extra virgin olive oil
- Juice of 1 lime
- 1 garlic clove, minced
- 1 teaspoon honey
- Salt and pepper to taste

Directions:

1. Place spiralized zucchini in a large bowl. Add cherry tomatoes, corn kernels, red onion, and avocado.

2. In a small bowl, whisk together olive oil, lime juice, minced garlic, honey, salt, and pepper to create the dressing.

3. Pour the dressing over the zucchini noodle mixture and toss gently to coat.

4. Garnish with chopped cilantro before serving.

5. Serve immediately or chill in the refrigerator for 30 minutes for flavors to combine.

Per serving: Calories: 250, Carbs: 20g, Fiber: 7g, Sugars: 9g, Protein: 4g, Saturated fat: 3g, Unsaturated fat: 14g

Difficulty rating: ★★☆☆☆

Roasted Brussels Sprouts with Balsamic Glaze

Servings: 4

Preparation time: 10 minutes

Cooking time: 25 minutes

Ingredients:

- 1 1/2 pounds Brussels sprouts, trimmed and halved
- 2 tablespoons olive oil
- Salt and pepper to taste
- 1/4 cup balsamic vinegar
- 2 tablespoons honey

Directions:

1. Preheat oven to 400°F (200°C).

2. In a large bowl, toss Brussels sprouts with olive oil, salt, and pepper until evenly coated.

3. Spread Brussels sprouts in a single layer on a baking sheet.

4. Roast in the preheated oven for 20-25 minutes, or until tender and caramelized, stirring halfway through.

5. While the Brussels sprouts are roasting, combine balsamic vinegar and honey in a small saucepan over medium heat.

6. Simmer until the mixture reduces by half and thickens into a glaze, about 5-7 minutes.

7. Drizzle the balsamic glaze over the roasted Brussels sprouts before serving.

Per serving: Calories: 180, Carbs: 24g, Fiber: 6g, Sugars: 12g, Protein: 6g, Saturated fat: 1g, Unsaturated fat: 7g

Difficulty rating: ★★☆☆☆

Grilled Asparagus with Lemon

Servings: 4

Preparation time: 5 minutes

Cooking time: 10 minutes

Ingredients:

- 1 pound asparagus, trimmed
- 2 tablespoons olive oil
- Salt and pepper to taste
- Juice of 1 lemon
- Lemon zest for garnish

Directions:

1. Preheat grill to medium-high heat.

2. Toss asparagus with olive oil, salt, and pepper in a bowl until evenly coated.

3. Grill asparagus for 2-3 minutes per side, or until tender and slightly charred.

4. Remove from grill and immediately drizzle with lemon juice.

5. Garnish with lemon zest before serving.

Per serving: Calories: 90, Carbs: 6g, Fiber: 3g, Sugars: 3g, Protein: 3g, Saturated fat: 1g, Unsaturated fat: 6g

Difficulty rating: ★☆☆☆☆

Purely Vegetarian

Cauliflower Steak with Turmeric Quinoa

Servings: 4

Preparation Time: 30 minutes

Cooking time: 20-25 minutes

Ingredients:

- 2 large heads of cauliflower, sliced into steaks
- 2 tablespoons olive oil
- 1 cup quinoa, cooked
- 1 teaspoon turmeric
- Salt and pepper to taste
- 1/4 cup pine nuts, toasted
- 1/4 cup parsley, chopped

Directions:

1. Preheat the oven to 400°F (200°C).

2. Brush cauliflower steaks with olive oil and season with salt and pepper. Place on a baking sheet.

3. Roast for 20-25 minutes, flipping halfway through, until golden and tender.

4. Mix cooked quinoa with turmeric, adding salt and pepper to taste.

5. Serve cauliflower steaks on a bed of turmeric quinoa, garnished with toasted pine nuts and chopped parsley.

Per serving: Calories: 310, Carbs: 35g, Fiber: 9g, Sugars: 6g, Protein: 10g, Saturated fat: 3g, Unsaturated fat: 8g

Difficulty rating: ★★☆☆☆

Eggplant and Lentil Bolognese

Servings: 4

Preparation Time: 45 minutes

Cooking time: 20 minutes

Ingredients:

- 1 large eggplant, diced
- 2 tablespoons olive oil
- 1 onion, chopped
- 2 cloves garlic, minced
- 1 cup green lentils, cooked
- 1 can (28 oz) crushed tomatoes
- 1 teaspoon oregano
- Salt and pepper to taste
- Fresh basil for garnish
- Whole grain spaghetti, cooked

Directions:

1. In a large skillet, heat olive oil over medium heat. Add eggplant, onion, and garlic, cooking until eggplant is soft.

2. Stir in cooked lentils, crushed tomatoes, and oregano. Season with salt and pepper.

3. Simmer for 20 minutes, or until the sauce has thickened.

4. Serve the bolognese over cooked whole grain spaghetti, garnished with fresh basil.

Per serving: Calories: 350, Carbs: 60g, Fiber: 15g, Sugars: 10g, Protein: 15g, Saturated fat: 1g, Unsaturated fat: 7g

Difficulty rating: ★★☆☆☆

Quinoa Stuffed Bell Peppers

Servings: 4

Preparation Time: 45 minutes

Cooking time: 45 minutes

Ingredients:

- 4 large bell peppers, halved and seeds removed
- 1 cup quinoa, cooked
- 1 can (15 oz) black beans, drained and rinsed
- 1 cup corn kernels, fresh or frozen
- 1/2 cup tomato sauce
- 1 teaspoon cumin
- 1 teaspoon smoked paprika
- Salt and pepper to taste
- 1/4 cup fresh cilantro, chopped
- 1 avocado, diced for garnish

Directions:

1. Preheat the oven to 375°F (190°C).

2. In a large bowl, mix together cooked quinoa, black beans, corn, tomato sauce, cumin, smoked paprika, salt, and pepper.

3. Arrange bell pepper halves in a baking dish, cut-side up.

4. Spoon the quinoa mixture into each bell pepper half, pressing down lightly to pack.

5. Cover the baking dish with aluminum foil and bake for 30 minutes.

6. Remove foil and bake for an additional 15 minutes, or until peppers are tender and filling is heated through.

7. Garnish with fresh cilantro and diced avocado before serving.

Per serving: Calories: 330, Carbs: 45g, Fiber: 13g, Sugars: 10g, Protein: 10g, Saturated fat: 1g, Unsaturated fat: 8g

Difficulty rating: ★★☆☆☆

Chickpea and Spinach Curry

Servings: 4

Preparation time: 10 minutes

Cooking time: 20 minutes

Ingredients:

- 2 tablespoons olive oil
- 1 large onion, finely chopped
- 3 cloves garlic, minced
- 1 tablespoon grated ginger
- 1 tablespoon curry powder
- 1 teaspoon ground turmeric
- 1 can (14 oz) diced tomatoes, undrained
- 1 can (15 oz) chickpeas, drained and rinsed
- 4 cups fresh spinach leaves
- 1 can (14 oz) coconut milk
- Salt and pepper to taste
- Fresh cilantro, for garnish
- Cooked rice, for serving

Directions:

1. Heat olive oil in a large skillet over medium heat. Add onion, garlic, and ginger, cooking until the onion is soft and translucent, about 5 minutes.

2. Stir in curry powder and turmeric, cooking for another minute until fragrant.

3. Add diced tomatoes with their juice and chickpeas to the skillet. Bring to a simmer and cook for 10 minutes.

4. Stir in spinach leaves and coconut milk, cooking until the spinach is wilted and the curry is heated through, about 5 minutes. Season with salt and pepper to taste.

5. Serve the curry over cooked rice, garnished with fresh cilantro.

Per serving: Calories: 350, Carbs: 40g, Fiber: 9g, Sugars: 8g, Protein: 10g, Saturated fat: 10g, Unsaturated fat: 5g

Difficulty rating: ★★☆☆☆

Sweet Potato and Chickpea Curry

Servings: 4

Preparation Time: 40 minutes

Cooking time: 25-30 minutes

Ingredients:

- 2 tablespoons coconut oil
- 1 onion, diced
- 2 cloves garlic, minced
- 1 tablespoon ginger, grated
- 1 large sweet potato, cubed
- 1 can (15 oz) chickpeas, drained and rinsed
- 1 can (14 oz) diced tomatoes
- 1 can (14 oz) coconut milk
- 2 teaspoons curry powder
- Salt and pepper to taste
- Fresh cilantro for garnish

Directions:

1. In a large pot, heat coconut oil over medium heat. Add onion, garlic, and ginger, cooking until onion is translucent.

2. Add sweet potato cubes, chickpeas, diced tomatoes, coconut milk, and curry powder. Stir to combine.

3. Bring to a boil, then reduce heat and simmer for 25-30 minutes, or until sweet potatoes are tender.

4. Season with salt and pepper to taste.

5. Garnish with fresh cilantro before serving.

Per serving: Calories: 450, Carbs: 55g, Fiber: 12g, Sugars: 12g, Protein: 12g, Saturated fat: 20g, Unsaturated fat: 5g

Difficulty rating: ★★☆☆☆

Creamy Mushroom and Spinach Pasta

Servings: 4

Preparation Time: 30 minutes

Cooking time: 15 minutes

Ingredients:

- 8 oz whole grain pasta
- 2 tablespoons olive oil
- 2 cloves garlic, minced
- 2 cups mushrooms, sliced
- 3 cups spinach leaves
- 1 cup coconut milk
- 1 teaspoon thyme
- Salt and pepper to taste
- Nutritional yeast for garnish

Directions:

1. Cook pasta according to package Directions; drain and set aside.

2. In a large skillet, heat olive oil over medium heat. Add garlic and mushrooms, sautéing until mushrooms are golden.

3. Add spinach and cook until wilted.

4. Pour in coconut milk and thyme, bringing to a simmer. Season with salt and pepper.

5. Add cooked pasta to the skillet, tossing to coat in the creamy sauce.

6. Serve sprinkled with nutritional yeast for a cheesy flavor.

Per serving: Calories: 340, Carbs: 45g, Fiber: 8g, Sugars: 3g, Protein: 10g, Saturated fat: 7g, Unsaturated fat: 8g

Difficulty rating: ★★☆☆☆

Stuffed Bell Peppers with Quinoa

Servings: 4

Preparation time: 15 minutes

Cooking time: 40 minutes

Ingredients:

- 4 large bell peppers, tops removed and seeded
- 1 cup quinoa, cooked
- 1 can (15 oz) black beans, drained and rinsed
- 1 cup corn kernels, fresh or frozen
- 1/2 cup tomato sauce
- 1 teaspoon cumin
- 1 teaspoon paprika
- 1/2 cup shredded vegan cheese
- Salt and pepper to taste
- Fresh cilantro, for garnish

Directions:

1. Preheat oven to 375°F (190°C).

2. In a bowl, mix together cooked quinoa, black beans, corn, tomato sauce, cumin, and paprika. Season with salt and pepper.

3. Stuff each bell pepper with the quinoa mixture and place in a baking dish.

4. Cover with foil and bake for 30 minutes. Remove foil, top each pepper with shredded vegan cheese, and bake for an additional 10 minutes, or until the cheese is melted and peppers are tender.

5. Serve hot, garnished with fresh cilantro.

Per serving: Calories: 280, Carbs: 50g, Fiber: 10g, Sugars: 8g, Protein: 12g, Saturated fat: 1g, Unsaturated fat: 2g

Difficulty rating: ★★☆☆☆

Vegan Mushroom Stroganoff

Servings: 4

Preparation time: 10 minutes

Cooking time: 20 minutes

Ingredients:

- 2 tablespoons olive oil
- 1 large onion, finely chopped
- 3 cloves garlic, minced
- 1 pound mushrooms, sliced
- 2 tablespoons all-purpose flour
- 2 cups vegetable broth
- 1 tablespoon soy sauce
- 1 teaspoon paprika
- 1 cup vegan sour cream
- Salt and pepper to taste
- Cooked pasta, for serving
- Fresh parsley, for garnish

Directions:

1. Heat olive oil in a large skillet over medium heat. Add onion and garlic, cooking until soft, about 5 minutes.

2. Add mushrooms and cook until they release their juices and become tender, about 8 minutes.

3. Sprinkle flour over the mushrooms and stir to combine. Cook for 2 minutes.

4. Gradually add vegetable broth and soy sauce, stirring constantly. Bring to a simmer and cook until the sauce thickens, about 5 minutes.

5. Stir in paprika and vegan sour cream. Season with salt and pepper to taste. Heat through, but do not boil.

6. Serve the stroganoff over cooked pasta, garnished with fresh parsley.

Per serving: Calories: 300, Carbs: 25g, Fiber: 3g, Sugars: 6g, Protein: 7g, Saturated fat: 2g, Unsaturated fat: 10g

Difficulty rating: ★★☆☆☆

Broccoli and Cashew Stir-Fry

Servings: 4

Preparation time: 15 minutes

Cooking time: 10 minutes

Ingredients:

- 2 tablespoons sesame oil
- 4 cups broccoli florets
- 1 red bell pepper, sliced
- 1 yellow bell pepper, sliced
- 2 cloves garlic, minced
- 1 tablespoon fresh ginger, grated
- 1/2 cup cashews, unsalted
- 2 tablespoons soy sauce
- 1 tablespoon maple syrup
- 1 tablespoon rice vinegar
- 1 teaspoon chili flakes (optional)
- Salt and pepper to taste
- Cooked brown rice, for serving

Directions:

1. Heat sesame oil in a large skillet or wok over medium-high heat. Add broccoli and bell peppers, stir-frying for about 5 minutes until vegetables are tender-crisp.

2. Add garlic and ginger, cooking for another minute until fragrant.

3. Stir in cashews, soy sauce, maple syrup, rice vinegar, and chili flakes if using. Cook for another 2-3 minutes, until the sauce thickens slightly and coats the vegetables.

4. Season with salt and pepper to taste.

5. Serve hot over cooked brown rice.

Per serving: Calories: 280, Carbs: 24g, Fiber: 4g, Sugars: 9g, Protein: 7g, Saturated fat: 2g, Unsaturated fat: 10g

Difficulty rating: ★★☆☆☆

Pumpkin and Chickpea Curry

Servings: 4

Preparation time: 15 minutes

Cooking time: 30 minutes

Ingredients:

- 2 cups pumpkin, peeled and cubed
- 1 can (15 oz) chickpeas, drained and rinsed
- 1 large onion, diced
- 2 cloves garlic, minced
- 1 tablespoon ginger, grated
- 1 can (14 oz) coconut milk
- 2 tablespoons curry powder
- 1 teaspoon turmeric
- 1 teaspoon cumin
- 1 tablespoon olive oil
- Salt and pepper to taste
- Fresh cilantro, for garnish

Directions:

1. Heat olive oil in a large skillet over medium heat. Add onion, garlic, and ginger, sautéing until onion is translucent, about 5 minutes.

2. Stir in curry powder, turmeric, and cumin, cooking for another minute until fragrant.

3. Add pumpkin cubes, chickpeas, and coconut milk to the skillet. Season with salt and pepper.

4. Bring to a simmer, cover, and cook for 25 minutes, or until pumpkin is tender.

5. Serve hot, garnished with fresh cilantro.

Per serving: Calories: 350, Carbs: 45g, Fiber: 10g, Sugars: 9g, Protein: 10g, Saturated fat: 15g, Unsaturated fat: 5g

Difficulty rating: ★★★★☆

Kale and Potato Hash

Servings: 4

Preparation time: 10 minutes

Cooking time: 20 minutes

Ingredients:

- 2 large potatoes, diced
- 2 cups kale, stems removed and chopped
- 1 medium onion, diced
- 2 cloves garlic, minced
- 2 tablespoons olive oil
- 1/2 teaspoon smoked paprika
- Salt and pepper to taste
- 4 eggs (optional, for serving on top)

Directions:

1. Heat olive oil in a large skillet over medium heat.

2. Add diced potatoes and cook for 10 minutes, stirring occasionally, until they start to soften.

3. Add diced onion and minced garlic to the skillet. Cook for another 5 minutes until onions are translucent.

4. Stir in chopped kale, smoked paprika, salt, and pepper. Cook until kale is wilted and potatoes are tender, about 5 more minutes.

5. In a separate pan, fry or poach eggs to your preference (optional).

6. Serve the hash in bowls, topped with an egg if using.

Per serving: (without egg): Calories: 250, Carbs: 35g, Fiber: 5g, Sugars: 3g, Protein: 5g, Saturated fat: 1g, Unsaturated fat: 9g

Difficulty rating: ★★☆☆☆

Beetroot and Lentil Burgers

Servings: 4

Preparation time: 20 minutes

Cooking time: 10 minutes

Ingredients:

- 1 cup cooked lentils
- 1 large beetroot, grated
- 1/2 cup breadcrumbs
- 1 small onion, finely chopped
- 2 cloves garlic, minced
- 1 teaspoon cumin
- 1/2 teaspoon smoked paprika
- Salt and pepper to taste
- 2 tablespoons olive oil, for frying
- Whole grain buns, for serving

Directions:

1. In a large bowl, mash the cooked lentils slightly with a fork.

2. Add grated beetroot, breadcrumbs, onion, garlic, cumin, smoked paprika, salt, and pepper. Mix until well combined.

3. Form the mixture into 4 patties.

4. Heat olive oil in a skillet over medium heat. Fry the patties for 5 minutes on each side, or until crispy and heated through.

5. Serve on whole grain buns with your favorite burger toppings.

Per serving: (burger only): Calories: 220, Carbs: 35g, Fiber: 8g, Sugars: 5g, Protein: 9g, Saturated fat: 1g, Unsaturated fat: 7g

Difficulty rating: ★★★☆☆

Cauliflower Tacos

Servings: 4

Preparation time: 15 minutes

Cooking time: 20 minutes

Ingredients:

- 1 head cauliflower, cut into small florets
- 2 tablespoons olive oil
- 1 teaspoon chili powder
- 1/2 teaspoon garlic powder
- 1/4 teaspoon cumin
- Salt and pepper to taste
- 8 small corn tortillas
- 1 avocado, sliced
- 1/4 cup red cabbage, shredded
- 1/4 cup fresh cilantro, chopped
- Lime wedges for serving
- 1/4 cup vegan sour cream (optional)

Directions:

1. Preheat oven to 400°F (200°C).

2. In a large bowl, toss cauliflower florets with olive oil, chili powder, garlic powder, cumin, salt, and pepper until well coated.

3. Spread cauliflower on a baking sheet in a single layer. Roast for 20 minutes, or until tender and slightly caramelized, stirring halfway through.

4. Warm corn tortillas in the oven for the last 5 minutes of cauliflower roasting time.

5. Assemble tacos by placing roasted cauliflower on tortillas, topped with avocado slices, shredded red cabbage, and cilantro.

6. Serve with lime wedges and vegan sour cream on the side, if desired.

Per serving: Calories: 280, Carbs: 35g, Fiber: 9g, Sugars: 4g, Protein: 6g, Saturated fat: 2g, Unsaturated fat: 10g

Difficulty rating: ★☆☆☆☆

Black Bean and Avocado Enchiladas

Servings: 4

Preparation time: 20 minutes

Cooking time: 25 minutes

Ingredients:

- 1 can (15 oz) black beans, drained and rinsed
- 2 avocados, diced
- 1/2 cup red onion, finely chopped
- 1/2 cup fresh cilantro, chopped
- Juice of 1 lime
- Salt and pepper to taste
- 8 corn tortillas
- 1 cup enchilada sauce
- 1 cup vegan cheese, shredded

Directions:

1. Preheat oven to 350°F (175°C).

2. In a bowl, combine black beans, diced avocados, red onion, cilantro, and lime juice. Season with salt and pepper to taste.

3. Soften corn tortillas by heating them in the microwave for 30 seconds or on a skillet for a few seconds on each side.

4. Spoon the black bean and avocado mixture evenly onto the center of each tortilla. Roll up and place seam-side down in a baking dish.

5. Pour enchilada sauce over the rolled tortillas and sprinkle with vegan cheese.

6. Bake in the preheated oven for 25 minutes, or until the cheese is melted and the enchiladas are heated through.

7. Serve hot.

Per serving: Calories: 350, Carbs: 45g, Fiber: 13g, Sugars: 5g, Protein: 12g, Saturated fat: 2g, Unsaturated fat: 10g

Difficulty rating: ★★☆☆☆

Butternut Squash Risotto

Servings: 4

Preparation time: 15 minutes

Cooking time: 30 minutes

Ingredients:

- 1 medium butternut squash, peeled and cubed
- 4 cups vegetable broth
- 1 tablespoon olive oil
- 1 small onion, finely chopped
- 2 cloves garlic, minced
- 1 cup Arborio rice
- 1/2 cup dry white wine
- Salt and pepper to taste
- 1/4 cup grated Parmesan cheese
- 2 tablespoons unsalted butter
- Fresh sage leaves for garnish

Directions:

1. In a saucepan, bring vegetable broth to a simmer. Add cubed butternut squash and cook until tender, about 10 minutes. Using a slotted spoon, transfer squash to a bowl and set aside. Keep broth warm over low heat.

2. In a large skillet, heat olive oil over medium heat. Add onion and garlic, sautéing until softened. Stir in Arborio rice, coating well with oil.

3. Pour in white wine, stirring constantly until the wine is absorbed.

4. Add warm broth one ladle at a time, stirring constantly until each ladle of broth is absorbed before adding the next. Continue until the rice is creamy and al dente, about 20 minutes.

5. Stir in cooked butternut squash, Parmesan cheese, and butter. Season with salt and pepper to taste.

6. Serve garnished with fresh sage leaves.

Per serving: Calories: 380, Carbs: 60g, Fiber: 4g, Sugars: 3g, Protein: 9g, Saturated fat: 5g, Unsaturated fat: 5g

Difficulty rating: ★★★☆☆

Spicy Tofu Stir-Fry

Servings: 4

Preparation time: 15 minutes

Cooking time: 10 minutes

Ingredients:

- 1 block (14 oz) firm tofu, pressed and cubed
- 2 tablespoons soy sauce
- 1 tablespoon sesame oil
- 1 tablespoon chili paste
- 2 cloves garlic, minced
- 1 inch ginger, grated
- 2 cups mixed bell peppers, sliced
- 1 cup broccoli florets
- 1/2 cup carrots, julienned
- 2 green onions, sliced
- 1 tablespoon sesame seeds
- Cooked rice, for serving

Directions:

1. In a bowl, toss tofu cubes with soy sauce. Let marinate for 10 minutes.

2. In a large skillet or wok, heat sesame oil over medium-high heat. Add chili paste, garlic, and ginger, sautéing for 1 minute.

3. Add marinated tofu to the skillet, cooking until browned on all sides.

4. Add bell peppers, broccoli, and carrots to the skillet. Stir-fry for 5 minutes, or until vegetables are tender-crisp.

5. Garnish with green onions and sesame seeds.

6. Serve hot over cooked rice.

Per serving: Calories: 220, Carbs: 18g, Fiber: 4g, Sugars: 6g, Protein: 14g, Saturated fat: 2g, Unsaturated fat: 7g

Difficulty rating: ★★☆☆☆

Eggplant Parmesan

Servings: 4

Preparation time: 15 minutes

Cooking time: 45 minutes

Ingredients:

- 2 large eggplants, sliced into 1/2 inch rounds
- 2 cups marinara sauce
- 2 cups shredded mozzarella cheese
- 1/2 cup grated Parmesan cheese
- 1/4 cup fresh basil leaves, chopped
- 2 eggs, beaten
- 1 cup breadcrumbs
- 1/2 cup all-purpose flour
- Salt and pepper to taste
- Olive oil for frying

Directions:

1. Preheat oven to 375°F (190°C).

2. Season eggplant slices with salt and let sit for 20 minutes to draw out moisture. Pat dry with paper towels.

3. Dredge eggplant slices in flour, dip in beaten eggs, then coat with breadcrumbs.

4. Heat olive oil in a skillet over medium heat. Fry eggplant slices until golden brown on both sides. Drain on paper towels.

5. Spread a thin layer of marinara sauce in the bottom of a baking dish. Layer eggplant slices, more sauce, mozzarella, and Parmesan cheese. Repeat layers, ending with cheese.

6. Bake in the preheated oven for 25 minutes, or until cheese is bubbly and golden.

7. Garnish with fresh basil before serving.

Per serving: Calories: 450, Carbs: 48g, Fiber: 9g, Sugars: 12g, Protein: 25g, Saturated fat: 10g, Unsaturated fat: 15g

Difficulty rating: ★★★☆☆

Quinoa Stuffed Tomatoes

Servings: 4

Preparation time: 20 minutes

Cooking time: 25 minutes

Ingredients:

- 4 large tomatoes
- 1 cup quinoa, cooked
- 1/2 cup black beans, drained and rinsed
- 1/2 cup corn kernels, fresh or thawed from frozen
- 1/4 cup red onion, finely chopped
- 1/4 cup cilantro, chopped
- 1 lime, juiced
- 1 teaspoon chili powder
- 1/2 teaspoon cumin
- Salt and pepper to taste
- 1/2 cup shredded cheddar cheese

Directions:

1. Preheat oven to 350°F (175°C).

2. Slice the tops off the tomatoes and scoop out the insides, leaving a shell.

3. In a bowl, mix together cooked quinoa, black beans, corn, red onion, cilantro, lime juice, chili powder, cumin, salt, and pepper.

4. Stuff the tomato shells with the quinoa mixture and place in a baking dish.

5. Top each tomato with shredded cheddar cheese.

6. Bake in the preheated oven for 20 minutes, or until tomatoes are tender and cheese is melted.

7. Serve hot as a main dish or a hearty side.

Per serving: Calories: 280, Carbs: 38g, Fiber: 7g, Sugars: 6g, Protein: 12g, Saturated fat: 4g, Unsaturated fat: 5g

Difficulty rating: ★★★★☆

Zucchini Lasagna

Servings: 6

Preparation time: 20 minutes

Cooking time: 45 minutes

Ingredients:

- 4 large zucchinis, sliced lengthwise into thin strips
- 1 tablespoon olive oil
- 1 small onion, diced
- 2 cloves garlic, minced
- 1 pound ground turkey
- 1 can (28 oz) crushed tomatoes
- 2 teaspoons dried oregano
- 1 teaspoon dried basil
- Salt and pepper to taste
- 1 cup ricotta cheese
- 1 egg
- 1/4 cup grated Parmesan cheese
- 2 cups shredded mozzarella cheese

Directions:

1. Preheat oven to 375°F (190°C). Grease a 9x13 inch baking dish.

2. In a skillet over medium heat, heat olive oil. Add onion and garlic, sautéing until softened. Add ground turkey, cooking until browned. Stir in crushed tomatoes, oregano, basil, salt, and pepper. Simmer for 10 minutes.

3. In a bowl, mix ricotta cheese, egg, and Parmesan cheese.

4. Lay zucchini strips in the baking dish to cover the bottom. Spread half of the turkey mixture over zucchini. Dollop half of the ricotta mixture on top, then sprinkle with 1 cup of mozzarella cheese. Repeat layers.

5. Cover with foil and bake for 30 minutes. Remove foil and bake another 15 minutes, or until cheese is golden and bubbly.

6. Let stand for 10 minutes before serving.

Per serving: Calories: 350, Carbs: 15g, Fiber: 3g, Sugars: 8g, Protein: 32g, Saturated fat: 9g, Unsaturated fat: 8g

Difficulty rating: ★★★☆☆

Moroccan Vegetable Tagine

Servings: 4

Preparation time: 20 minutes

Cooking time: 40 minutes

Ingredients:

- 2 tablespoons olive oil
- 1 large onion, finely chopped
- 2 cloves garlic, minced
- 1 teaspoon ground cumin
- 1 teaspoon ground cinnamon
- 1/2 teaspoon ground turmeric
- 1/4 teaspoon cayenne pepper
- 1 can (14.5 oz) undrained diced tomatoes
- 1 cup vegetable broth
- 2 carrots, peeled and sliced
- 2 cups cubed butternut squash (peeled)
- 1 zucchini, sliced
- 1 bell pepper, chopped
- 1 cup chickpeas, drained and rinsed
- 1/2 cup dried apricots, chopped
- Salt and pepper to taste
- Fresh cilantro, for garnish

Directions:

1. Heat olive oil in a large pot or tagine over medium heat. Add onion and garlic, cooking until softened, about 5 minutes.

2. Stir in cumin, cinnamon, turmeric, and cayenne pepper, cooking for another minute until fragrant.

3. Add diced tomatoes, vegetable broth, carrots, butternut squash, zucchini, bell pepper, chickpeas, and dried apricots.

4. Bring to a boil, then reduce heat, cover, and simmer for 35 minutes, or until vegetables are tender.

5. Serve hot, garnished with fresh cilantro.

Per serving: Calories: 260, Carbs: 45g, Fiber: 9g, Sugars: 20g, Protein: 7g, Saturated fat: 1g, Unsaturated fat: 7g

Difficulty rating: ★★☆☆☆

Vegan Paella

Servings: 4

Preparation time: 20 minutes

Cooking time: 40 minutes

Ingredients:

- 2 tablespoons olive oil
- 1 large onion, diced
- 2 cloves garlic, minced
- 1 red bell pepper, diced
- 1 yellow bell pepper, diced
- 1 cup short-grain brown rice
- 1 teaspoon turmeric
- 1/2 teaspoon smoked paprika
- 1/4 teaspoon cayenne pepper
- 3 cups vegetable broth
- 1 can (14 oz) diced tomatoes, undrained
- 1 cup frozen green peas
- 1 cup artichoke hearts, quartered
- Salt and pepper to taste
- Lemon wedges, for serving
- Fresh parsley, chopped, for garnish

Directions:

1. Heat olive oil in a large skillet or paella pan over medium heat. Add onion and garlic, sautéing until softened, about 5 minutes.

2. Add both bell peppers and cook for another 5 minutes, until slightly softened.

3. Stir in rice, turmeric, smoked paprika, and cayenne pepper until the rice is well coated with the spices.

4. Pour in vegetable broth and diced tomatoes with their juice. Bring to a simmer, then reduce heat to low. Cover and cook for 30 minutes, or until rice is almost tender.

5. Stir in green peas and artichoke hearts. Season with salt and pepper. Cover and cook for an additional 10 minutes.

6. Remove from heat and let sit, covered, for 5 minutes before serving.

7. Serve with lemon wedges and garnish with fresh parsley.

Per serving: Calories: 320, Carbs: 58g, Fiber: 8g, Sugars: 9g, Protein: 9g, Saturated fat: 1g, Unsaturated fat: 7g

Difficulty rating: ★★☆☆☆

Sweet Potato and Black Bean Chili

Servings: 4

Preparation time: 15 minutes

Cooking time: 35 minutes

Ingredients:

- 2 tablespoons olive oil
- 1 large sweet potato, peeled and diced
- 1 large onion, diced
- 3 cloves garlic, minced
- 2 tablespoons chili powder
- 1 tablespoon ground cumin
- 1/4 teaspoon ground chipotle pepper
- 3 cups vegetable broth
- 1 can (15 oz) black beans, drained and rinsed
- 1 can (14.5 oz) diced tomatoes
- 1/2 cup quinoa
- Salt and pepper to taste
- Avocado slices, for garnish
- Fresh cilantro, chopped, for garnish

Directions:

1. Heat olive oil in a large pot over medium heat. Add sweet potato and onion, cooking until the onion is translucent, about 5 minutes.

2. Add garlic, chili powder, cumin, and chipotle pepper, stirring for about 1 minute until fragrant.

3. Pour in vegetable broth, black beans, and diced tomatoes with their juice. Bring to a boil.

4. Stir in quinoa, then reduce heat to low. Cover and simmer for 25 minutes, or until the sweet potato is tender and the quinoa is cooked.

5. Season with salt and pepper to taste.

6. Serve hot, garnished with avocado slices and chopped cilantro.

Per serving: Calories: 330, Carbs: 55g, Fiber: 13g, Sugars: 8g, Protein: 12g, Saturated fat: 1g, Unsaturated fat: 7g

Difficulty rating: ★★☆☆☆

Meat & Poultry Favorites

Rosemary Lemon Chicken Skewers

Servings: 4

Preparation Time: 25 minutes

Cooking time: 10-12 minutes

Ingredients:

- 1 pound chicken breast, cut into 1-inch pieces
- 2 tablespoons olive oil
- 2 tablespoons fresh rosemary, finely chopped
- Zest and juice of 1 lemon
- 2 cloves garlic, minced
- Salt and pepper to taste
- 1 bell pepper, cut into 1-inch pieces
- 1 red onion, cut into 1-inch pieces

Directions:

1. In a bowl, whisk together olive oil, rosemary, lemon zest, lemon juice, garlic, salt, and pepper.

2. Add chicken pieces to the marinade, ensuring they are well coated. Let marinate for at least 15 minutes, or up to 2 hours in the refrigerator.

3. Preheat grill to medium-high heat.

4. Thread marinated chicken pieces onto skewers, alternating with bell pepper and red onion pieces.

5. Grill skewers, turning occasionally, until chicken is cooked through and vegetables are slightly charred, about 10-12 minutes.

6. Serve hot, garnished with additional fresh rosemary and lemon wedges if desired.

Per serving: Calories: 250, Carbs: 5g, Fiber: 1g, Sugars: 2g, Protein: 25g, Saturated fat: 2g, Unsaturated fat: 7g

Difficulty rating: ★★☆☆☆

Turmeric Ginger Turkey Burgers

Servings: 4

Preparation Time: 20 minutes

Cooking time: 10-14 minutes

Ingredients:

- 1 pound ground turkey
- 1 teaspoon ground turmeric
- 1 teaspoon fresh ginger, grated
- 1/4 cup fresh cilantro, finely chopped
- 1 green onion, finely chopped
- Salt and pepper to taste
- 1 tablespoon olive oil
- Whole grain buns, for serving
- Lettuce, tomato, and avocado slices for garnish

Directions:

1. In a large bowl, combine ground turkey, turmeric, ginger, cilantro, green onion, salt, and pepper. Mix until well combined.

2. Form the mixture into 4 patties.

3. Heat olive oil in a skillet over medium heat. Cook patties for 5-7 minutes on each side, or until fully cooked and golden brown.

4. Serve the turkey burgers on whole grain buns, topped with lettuce, tomato, and avocado slices.

Per serving: Calories: 310, Carbs: 23g, Fiber: 3g, Sugars: 4g, Protein: 28g, Saturated fat: 2g, Unsaturated fat: 8g

Difficulty rating: ★★☆☆☆

Balsamic Glazed Pork Tenderloin

Servings: 4

Preparation Time: 30 minutes

Cooking time: 15-20 minutes

Ingredients:

- 1 pork tenderloin (about 1 pound)
- Salt and pepper to taste
- 2 tablespoons olive oil
- 1/4 cup balsamic vinegar
- 2 tablespoons honey
- 1 teaspoon fresh thyme, chopped
- 2 cloves garlic, minced

Directions:

1. Preheat oven to 375°F (190°C).

2. Season pork tenderloin with salt and pepper.

3. Heat olive oil in an oven-safe skillet over medium-high heat. Sear the tenderloin on all sides until golden brown.

4. In a small bowl, whisk together balsamic vinegar, honey, thyme, and garlic. Pour over the seared tenderloin.

5. Transfer the skillet to the oven and roast for 15-20 minutes, or until a thermometer inserted into the thickest part reads 145°F (63°C).

6. Let the tenderloin rest for 5 minutes before slicing. Serve drizzled with the balsamic glaze from the pan.

Per serving: Calories: 290, Carbs: 15g, Fiber: 0g, Sugars: 12g, Protein: 28g, Saturated fat: 2g, Unsaturated fat: 10g

Difficulty rating: ★★☆☆☆

Spiced Beef and Vegetable Stir-Fry

Servings: 4

Preparation Time: 20 minutes

Cooking time: 8-10 minutes

Ingredients:

- 1 pound lean beef, thinly sliced
- 2 tablespoons soy sauce (gluten-free if necessary)
- 1 tablespoon sesame oil
- 1 teaspoon ground cumin
- 1 teaspoon ground coriander
- 2 cups broccoli florets
- 1 red bell pepper, sliced
- 1 carrot, julienned
- 2 cloves garlic, minced
- 1 tablespoon fresh ginger, grated
- 1 tablespoon olive oil

Directions:

1. In a bowl, marinate beef slices with soy sauce, sesame oil, cumin, and coriander for at least 10 minutes.

2. Heat olive oil in a large skillet or wok over high heat. Add garlic and ginger, sautéing for 30 seconds.

3. Add marinated beef and stir-fry until browned, about 3-4 minutes.

4. Add broccoli, bell pepper, and carrot to the skillet. Continue to stir-fry until vegetables are tender-crisp, about 5 minutes.

5. Serve hot, garnished with sesame seeds if desired.

Per serving: Calories: 280, Carbs: 10g, Fiber: 3g, Sugars: 4g, Protein: 26g, Saturated fat: 3g, Unsaturated fat: 7g

Difficulty rating: ★★☆☆☆

Grilled Chicken with Rosemary and Lemon

Servings: 4

Preparation time: 15 minutes

Cooking time: 20 minutes

Ingredients:

- 4 boneless, skinless chicken breasts
- 2 tablespoons olive oil
- Juice of 1 lemon
- 2 garlic cloves, minced
- 2 tablespoons fresh rosemary, chopped
- Salt and pepper to taste

Directions:

1. In a small bowl, whisk together olive oil, lemon juice, minced garlic, chopped rosemary, salt, and pepper.

2. Place chicken breasts in a shallow dish and pour the marinade over them. Ensure each piece is well coated. Cover and refrigerate for at least 1 hour.

3. Preheat grill to medium-high heat.

4. Remove chicken from marinade, letting excess drip off. Grill chicken for 10 minutes on each side or until internal temperature reaches 165°F (74°C).

5. Serve hot, garnished with lemon slices and additional rosemary if desired.

Per serving: Calories: 220, Carbs: 2g, Fiber: 0g, Sugars: 0g, Protein: 26g, Saturated fat: 2g, Unsaturated fat: 10g

Difficulty rating: ★★☆☆☆

Baked Salmon with Dill and Lemon

Servings: 4

Preparation time: 10 minutes

Cooking time: 15 minutes

Ingredients:

- 4 salmon fillets (6 ounces each)
- 2 tablespoons olive oil
- Juice of 1 lemon
- 2 tablespoons fresh dill, chopped
- Salt and pepper to taste
- Lemon slices for garnish

Directions:

1. Preheat oven to 400°F (200°C). Line a baking sheet with parchment paper.

2. Place salmon fillets on the prepared baking sheet. Drizzle with olive oil and lemon juice. Sprinkle with chopped dill, salt, and pepper.

3. Bake in the preheated oven for 12-15 minutes, or until salmon flakes easily with a fork.

4. Serve hot, garnished with lemon slices and additional dill if desired.

Per serving: Calories: 280, Carbs: 1g, Fiber: 0g, Sugars: 0g, Protein: 23g, Saturated fat: 4g, Unsaturated fat: 13g

Difficulty rating: ★☆☆☆☆

Turkey and Quinoa Meatballs

Servings: 4

Preparation time: 20 minutes

Cooking time: 25 minutes

Ingredients:

- 1 pound ground turkey
- 1 cup cooked quinoa
- 1 egg, beaten
- 1/4 cup onion, finely chopped
- 2 cloves garlic, minced
- 2 tablespoons fresh parsley, chopped
- 1 teaspoon dried oregano
- Salt and pepper to taste
- 1/2 cup marinara sauce for serving

Directions:

1. Preheat oven to 375°F (190°C). Line a baking sheet with parchment paper.

2. In a large bowl, combine ground turkey, cooked quinoa, beaten egg, chopped onion, minced garlic, chopped parsley, dried oregano, salt, and pepper. Mix until well combined.

3. Form the mixture into 1-inch meatballs and place on the prepared baking sheet.

4. Bake in the preheated oven for 20-25 minutes, or until meatballs are cooked through and lightly golden.

5. Serve hot with marinara sauce on the side.

Per serving: Calories: 240, Carbs: 15g, Fiber: 2g, Sugars: 2g, Protein: 27g, Saturated fat: 1g, Unsaturated fat: 3g

Difficulty rating: ★★☆☆☆

Stir-Fried Beef with Broccoli and Ginger

Servings: 4

Preparation time: 15 minutes

Cooking time: 10 minutes

Ingredients:

- 1 lb beef sirloin, thinly sliced
- 4 cups broccoli florets
- 2 tablespoons olive oil
- 3 cloves garlic, minced
- 2 inches fresh ginger, peeled and grated
- 1/4 cup soy sauce
- 2 tablespoons oyster sauce
- 1 tablespoon honey
- 1 teaspoon sesame oil
- Salt and pepper to taste
- Sesame seeds for garnish

Directions:

1. Heat 1 tablespoon of olive oil in a large skillet or wok over medium-high heat. Add garlic and ginger, sautéing until fragrant, about 1 minute.

2. Add the sliced beef to the skillet, seasoning with a pinch of salt and pepper. Stir-fry until the beef is browned and cooked through, about 3-4 minutes. Remove beef from the skillet and set aside.

3. In the same skillet, add the remaining tablespoon of olive oil and broccoli florets. Stir-fry until the broccoli is bright green and tender-crisp, about 4-5 minutes.

4. Return the beef to the skillet. Add soy sauce, oyster sauce, honey, and sesame oil. Stir well to combine and cook for an additional 2 minutes.

5. Serve hot, garnished with sesame seeds.

Per serving: Calories: 320, Carbs: 15g, Fiber: 3g, Sugars: 6g, Protein: 25g, Saturated fat: 4g, Unsaturated fat: 8g

Difficulty rating: ★★☆☆☆

Pork Tenderloin with Apple Cider Glaze

Servings: 4

Preparation time: 10 minutes

Cooking time: 25 minutes

Ingredients:

- 1 lb pork tenderloin
- Salt and pepper to taste
- 2 tablespoons olive oil
- 1/2 cup apple cider
- 2 tablespoons honey
- 2 tablespoons Dijon mustard
- 1 tablespoon apple cider vinegar
- 1 teaspoon fresh rosemary, finely chopped

Directions:

1. Preheat oven to 375°F (190°C). Season the pork tenderloin with salt and pepper.

2. Heat olive oil in an oven-safe skillet over medium-high heat. Add the pork tenderloin and sear on all sides until golden brown, about 2-3 minutes per side.

3. In a small bowl, whisk together apple cider, honey, Dijon mustard, and apple cider vinegar. Pour the mixture over the pork in the skillet.

4. Place the skillet in the preheated oven and roast for 15-20 minutes, or until the pork reaches an internal temperature of 145°F (63°C).

5. Remove from oven and let the pork rest for 5 minutes. Slice and drizzle with the apple cider glaze from the skillet. Garnish with fresh rosemary.

Per serving: Calories: 280, Carbs: 15g, Fiber: 0g, Sugars: 12g, Protein: 24g, Saturated fat: 3g, Unsaturated fat: 5g

Difficulty rating: ★★☆☆

Chicken Curry with Turmeric and Coconut Milk

Servings: 4

Preparation time: 15 minutes

Cooking time: 30 minutes

Ingredients:

- 1 lb chicken breast, cut into bite-sized pieces
- 2 tablespoons coconut oil
- 1 large onion, diced
- 3 cloves garlic, minced
- 1 tablespoon fresh ginger, grated
- 1 tablespoon ground turmeric
- 1 teaspoon ground cumin
- 1 teaspoon ground coriander
- 1 can (14 oz) coconut milk
- 1 cup chicken broth
- 1 tablespoon tomato paste
- Salt and pepper to taste
- Fresh cilantro, for garnish
- Cooked rice, for serving

Directions:

1. Heat coconut oil in a large skillet over medium heat. Add onion, garlic, and ginger, cooking until the onion is translucent, about 5 minutes.

2. Stir in turmeric, cumin, and coriander, cooking for another minute until fragrant.

3. Add chicken pieces to the skillet, seasoning with salt and pepper. Cook until the chicken is browned on all sides, about 5-7 minutes.

4. Pour in coconut milk, chicken broth, and tomato paste. Stir well to combine. Bring to a simmer, then reduce heat and cover. Cook for 20 minutes, or until the chicken is tender and the sauce has thickened.

5. Serve hot over cooked rice, garnished with fresh cilantro.

Per serving: Calories: 350, Carbs: 8g, Fiber: 1g, Sugars: 3g, Protein: 26g, Saturated fat: 14g, Unsaturated fat: 4g

Difficulty rating: ★★☆☆

Lemon and Thyme Roasted Chicken

Servings: 4

Preparation time: 15 minutes

Cooking time: 1 hour 20 minutes

Ingredients:

- 1 (4 to 5 lb) whole chicken
- 2 tablespoons olive oil
- 1 lemon, halved
- 4 sprigs fresh thyme
- Salt and pepper to taste
- 1 onion, quartered
- 4 cloves garlic, smashed

Directions:

1. Preheat oven to 425°F (220°C).

2. Rub the chicken all over with olive oil. Squeeze the juice of one lemon half inside the cavity and the other half over the outside of the chicken. Season the chicken inside and out with salt and pepper. Place thyme sprigs inside the cavity.

3. In a roasting pan, scatter the onion quarters and garlic cloves. Place the chicken breast side up on top of the onions and garlic.

4. Roast in the preheated oven for 1 hour and 20 minutes, or until the juices run clear when you cut between a leg and thigh.

5. Remove from oven and let rest for 10 minutes before carving.

6. Serve hot, garnished with additional fresh thyme if desired.

Per serving: Calories: 410, Carbs: 5g, Fiber: 1g, Sugars: 2g, Protein: 35g, Saturated fat: 9g, Unsaturated fat: 15g

Difficulty rating: ★★☆☆☆

Turkey Chili with Sweet Potatoes

Servings: 6

Preparation time: 15 minutes

Cooking time: 45 minutes

Ingredients:

- 2 tablespoons olive oil
- 1 lb ground turkey
- 1 large onion, diced
- 3 cloves garlic, minced
- 2 medium sweet potatoes, peeled and cubed
- 1 can (15 oz) black beans, drained and rinsed
- 1 can (28 oz) diced tomatoes, undrained
- 2 cups chicken broth
- 2 tablespoons chili powder
- 1 tablespoon ground cumin
- 1 teaspoon smoked paprika
- Salt and pepper to taste
- Fresh cilantro, for garnish
- Avocado slices, for garnish

Directions:

1. Heat olive oil in a large pot over medium heat. Add ground turkey, onion, and garlic. Cook until turkey is browned and onions are soft, about 10 minutes.

2. Add sweet potatoes, black beans, diced tomatoes with their juice, chicken broth, chili powder, cumin, and smoked paprika. Season with salt and pepper.

3. Bring to a boil, then reduce heat to low and simmer, covered, for 30 minutes, or until sweet potatoes are tender.

4. Serve hot, garnished with fresh cilantro and avocado slices.

Per serving: Calories: 320, Carbs: 35g, Fiber: 8g, Sugars: 9g, Protein: 22g, Saturated fat: 2g, Unsaturated fat: 5g

Difficulty rating: ★★☆☆☆

Baked Cod with Parsley and Olive Oil

Servings: 4

Preparation time: 10 minutes

Cooking time: 15 minutes

Ingredients:

- 4 cod fillets (6 ounces each)
- 4 tablespoons olive oil
- 1/4 cup fresh parsley, finely chopped
- 2 cloves garlic, minced
- Juice of 1 lemon
- Salt and pepper to taste
- Lemon wedges, for serving

Directions:

1. Preheat oven to 400°F (200°C). Line a baking sheet with parchment paper.

2. Place cod fillets on the prepared baking sheet. Drizzle each fillet with 1 tablespoon of olive oil.

3. In a small bowl, mix together parsley, garlic, and lemon juice. Spoon the mixture over the cod fillets. Season with salt and pepper.

4. Bake in the preheated oven for 12-15 minutes, or until the fish flakes easily with a fork.

5. Serve immediately with lemon wedges on the side.

Per serving: Calories: 200, Carbs: 1g, Fiber: 0g, Sugars: 0g, Protein: 23g, Saturated fat: 1g, Unsaturated fat: 13g

Difficulty rating: ★☆☆☆☆

Grilled Pork Chops with Peach Salsa

Servings: 4

Preparation time: 20 minutes (plus marinating time)

Cooking time: 12 minutes

Ingredients:

- 4 pork chops, bone-in (about 1 inch thick)
- 2 tablespoons olive oil
- Salt and pepper to taste

For the Peach Salsa:

- 2 ripe peaches, diced
- 1/4 cup red onion, finely chopped
- 1 jalapeño, seeded and minced
- 1/4 cup fresh cilantro, chopped
- Juice of 1 lime
- Salt to taste

Directions:

1. Preheat grill to medium-high heat.

2. Rub pork chops with olive oil and season with salt and pepper. Let marinate for at least 30 minutes in the refrigerator.

3. In a bowl, combine diced peaches, red onion, jalapeño, cilantro, and lime juice. Season with salt and mix well. Set aside to let flavors meld.

4. Grill pork chops for 5-6 minutes per side, or until the internal temperature reaches 145°F (63°C).

5. Remove pork chops from the grill and let rest for 5 minutes.

6. Serve pork chops topped with peach salsa.

Per serving: Calories: 310, Carbs: 9g, Fiber: 2g, Sugars: 6g, Protein: 35g, Saturated fat: 5g, Unsaturated fat: 15g

Difficulty rating: ★★☆☆☆

Beef and Broccoli Stir-Fry

Servings: 4

Preparation time: 15 minutes

Cooking time: 10 minutes

Ingredients:

- 1 lb beef sirloin, thinly sliced
- 4 cups broccoli florets
- 2 tablespoons olive oil
- 2 cloves garlic, minced
- 1 tablespoon fresh ginger, grated
- 1/4 cup soy sauce
- 2 tablespoons water
- 1 tablespoon cornstarch
- 1 tablespoon honey
- 1 teaspoon sesame oil
- Salt and pepper to taste
- Sesame seeds for garnish

Directions:

1. In a small bowl, whisk together soy sauce, water, cornstarch, honey, and sesame oil. Set aside.

2. Heat olive oil in a large skillet over medium-high heat. Add garlic and ginger, sautéing until fragrant, about 1 minute.

3. Add beef to the skillet, seasoning with salt and pepper. Cook until browned, about 3-4 minutes.

4. Add broccoli to the skillet, stirring to combine. Cook until broccoli is bright green and tender, about 3 minutes.

5. Pour the soy sauce mixture over the beef and broccoli. Stir well to coat and continue cooking until the sauce has thickened, about 2 minutes.

6. Serve hot, garnished with sesame seeds.

Per serving: Calories: 280, Carbs: 15g, Fiber: 3g, Sugars: 6g, Protein: 25g, Saturated fat: 3g, Unsaturated fat: 9g

Difficulty rating: ★★☆☆☆

Spicy Shrimp with Garlic and Herbs

Servings: 4

Preparation time: 10 minutes

Cooking time: 5 minutes

Ingredients:

- 1 lb large shrimp, peeled and deveined
- 3 tablespoons olive oil
- 4 cloves garlic, minced
- 1 teaspoon red pepper flakes
- 1 teaspoon paprika
- 1 tablespoon lemon juice
- 2 tablespoons fresh parsley, chopped
- Salt and pepper to taste

Directions:

1. In a large skillet, heat olive oil over medium-high heat. Add garlic and red pepper flakes, cooking until fragrant, about 1 minute.

2. Add shrimp to the skillet, seasoning with paprika, salt, and pepper. Cook until shrimp are pink and opaque, about 2-3 minutes per side.

3. Remove from heat and stir in lemon juice and fresh parsley.

4. Serve immediately.

Per serving: Calories: 220, Carbs: 2g, Fiber: 0g, Sugars: 0g, Protein: 24g, Saturated fat: 1g, Unsaturated fat: 9g

Difficulty rating: ★☆☆☆☆

Chicken Fajitas with Bell Peppers

Servings: 4

Preparation time: 15 minutes

Cooking time: 20 minutes

Ingredients:

- 1 1/2 pounds chicken breast, thinly sliced
- 2 tablespoons olive oil, divided
- 1 tablespoon chili powder
- 1 teaspoon cumin
- 1/2 teaspoon smoked paprika
- 1/2 teaspoon garlic powder
- Salt and pepper to taste
- 1 red bell pepper, sliced
- 1 green bell pepper, sliced
- 1 yellow bell pepper, sliced
- 1 large onion, sliced
- 8 flour tortillas, warmed
- Lime wedges, for serving
- Fresh cilantro, for garnish

Directions:

1. In a large bowl, combine chicken slices with 1 tablespoon olive oil, chili powder, cumin, smoked paprika, garlic powder, salt, and pepper. Toss to coat evenly.

2. Heat the remaining tablespoon of olive oil in a large skillet over medium-high heat. Add chicken and cook for 5-7 minutes, or until fully cooked. Remove chicken from skillet and set aside.

3. In the same skillet, add sliced bell peppers and onion. Cook for 5-8 minutes, or until vegetables are tender and slightly charred.

4. Return the cooked chicken to the skillet with the vegetables and stir to combine. Cook for an additional 2 minutes.

5. Serve chicken and vegetable mixture on warmed flour tortillas, garnished with lime wedges and fresh cilantro.

Per serving: Calories: 450, Carbs: 35g, Fiber: 3g, Sugars: 5g, Protein: 40g, Saturated fat: 2g, Unsaturated fat: 10g

Difficulty rating: ★★☆☆☆

Beef Stew with Root Vegetables

Servings: 6

Preparation time: 20 minutes

Cooking time: 2 hours

Ingredients:

- 2 lbs beef chuck, cut into 1-inch pieces
- 3 tablespoons olive oil
- 1 large onion, chopped
- 3 cloves garlic, minced
- 4 carrots, peeled and cut into 1-inch pieces
- 3 parsnips, peeled cut into 1-inch pieces
- 2 turnips, peeled and cut into 1-inch pieces
- 4 cups beef broth
- 1 cup red wine
- 2 tablespoons tomato paste
- 1 teaspoon dried thyme
- 1 teaspoon dried rosemary
- Salt and pepper to taste
- 2 tablespoons all-purpose flour
- Fresh parsley, chopped for garnish

Directions:

1. Heat 2 tablespoons olive oil in a large pot over medium-high heat. Season beef with salt and pepper. Add beef to the pot and brown on all sides. Remove beef and set aside.

2. In the same pot, add the remaining tablespoon of olive oil, onion, and garlic. Cook until softened, about 5 minutes.

3. Stir in tomato paste, thyme, and rosemary. Cook for 1 minute.

4. Add beef broth, red wine, carrots, parsnips, and turnips. Return beef to the pot. Bring to a boil, then reduce heat to low, cover, and simmer for 1.5 hours, or until beef is tender.

5. In a small bowl, mix flour with 2 tablespoons of water to make a paste. Stir into stew to thicken. Simmer for an additional 10 minutes.

6. Season with salt and pepper to taste. Serve hot, garnished with fresh parsley.

Per serving: Calories: 450, Carbs: 22g, Fiber: 5g, Sugars: 8g, Protein: 35g, Saturated fat: 10g, Unsaturated fat: 15g

Difficulty rating: ★★★☆☆

Seafood Selections

Lemon Herb Poached Salmon

Servings: 4

Preparation time: 10 minutes

Cooking time: 15 minutes

Ingredients:

- 4 salmon fillets (6 ounces each)
- 4 cups water
- 1 lemon, sliced
- 2 garlic cloves, minced
- 2 tablespoons fresh dill, chopped
- Salt and pepper to taste

Directions:

1. In a large skillet or saucepan, combine water, lemon slices, and garlic. Bring to a simmer over medium heat.

2. Season salmon fillets with salt and pepper, then place them in the simmering water. Ensure the water covers the fillets.

3. Poach the salmon gently until cooked through, about 12-15 minutes.

4. Remove from the water, garnish with fresh dill, and serve immediately.

Per serving: Calories: 300, Carbs: 1g, Fiber: 0g, Sugars: 0g, Protein: 34g, Saturated fat: 2g, Unsaturated fat: 12g

Difficulty rating: ★★☆☆☆

Grilled Mackerel with Orange and Fennel

Servings: 4

Preparation time: 15 minutes

Cooking time: 10 minutes

Ingredients:

- 4 mackerel fillets
- 2 tablespoons olive oil
- 1 fennel bulb, thinly sliced
- 1 orange, segmented
- 1 tablespoon orange zest
- Salt and pepper to taste

Directions:

1. Preheat the grill to medium-high heat.

2. Brush mackerel fillets with olive oil and season with salt and pepper.

3. Grill the fillets skin-side down for about 5-6 minutes, then flip carefully and cook for another 4 minutes or until cooked through.

4. In a bowl, toss the fennel slices, orange segments, and orange zest.

5. Serve the grilled mackerel topped with the fennel and orange salad.

Per serving: Calories: 290, Carbs: 10g, Fiber: 3g, Sugars: 6g, Protein: 25g, Saturated fat: 5g, Unsaturated fat: 15g

Difficulty rating: ★★☆☆☆

Baked Sardines with Lemon and Herbs

Servings: 4

Preparation time: 10 minutes

Cooking time: 15 minutes

Ingredients:

- 16 fresh sardines, cleaned and gutted
- 4 tablespoons olive oil
- 2 lemons, one sliced and one juiced
- 2 tablespoons chopped parsley
- 2 cloves garlic, minced
- Salt and pepper to taste

Directions:

1. Preheat the oven to 375°F (190°C).

2. Arrange sardines in a single layer in a baking dish. Drizzle with olive oil and lemon juice. Season with salt and pepper.

3. Scatter garlic, parsley, and lemon slices over the sardines.

4. Bake in the preheated oven until the sardines are cooked through, about 12-15 minutes.

5. Serve hot, garnished with additional parsley if desired.

Per serving: Calories: 250, Carbs: 2g, Fiber: 0g, Sugars: 0g, Protein: 34g, Saturated fat: 3g, Unsaturated fat: 10g

Difficulty rating: ★☆☆☆☆

Herbed Salmon and Asparagus Foil Packets

Servings: 4

Preparation time: 10 minutes

Cooking time: 20 minutes

Ingredients:

- 4 salmon fillets (6 ounces each)
- 1 bunch asparagus, trimmed
- 2 tablespoons olive oil
- 1 lemon, thinly sliced
- 2 tablespoons fresh dill, chopped
- Salt and pepper to taste

Directions:

1. Preheat your oven to 400°F (200°C).

2. Cut four sheets of aluminum foil, large enough to wrap a salmon fillet and a portion of asparagus.

3. Place a salmon fillet and a quarter of the asparagus in the center of each foil sheet.

4. Drizzle with olive oil and season with salt and pepper. Top with lemon slices and sprinkle with dill.

5. Fold the foil over the salmon and asparagus, sealing all edges to create a packet.

6. Bake for 20 minutes or until salmon is cooked through and asparagus is tender.

7. Serve immediately, opening the packets carefully to release steam.

Per serving: Calories: 310, Carbs: 5g, Fiber: 2g, Sugars: 2g, Protein: 34g, Saturated fat: 3g, Unsaturated fat: 10g

Difficulty rating: ★☆☆☆☆

Chili-Lime Shrimp Tacos

Servings: 4

Preparation time: 15 minutes

Cooking time: 5 minutes

Ingredients:

- 1 lb large shrimp, peeled and deveined
- 2 tablespoons olive oil
- Juice and zest of 1 lime
- 1 teaspoon chili powder
- 1/2 teaspoon garlic powder
- 8 small corn tortillas
- 1 avocado, sliced
- 1/4 cup fresh cilantro, chopped
- Salt and pepper to taste

Directions:

1. In a bowl, mix olive oil, lime juice and zest, chili powder, and garlic powder. Add shrimp and toss to coat.

2. Heat a large skillet over medium-high heat. Add shrimp and cook until pink and opaque, about 2-3 minutes per side.

3. Warm tortillas according to package Directions.

4. Assemble tacos by placing shrimp on tortillas, topped with avocado slices and cilantro.

5. Serve immediately with lime wedges on the side.

Per serving: Calories: 290, Carbs: 18g, Fiber: 5g, Sugars: 2g, Protein: 25g, Saturated fat: 2g, Unsaturated fat: 10g

Difficulty rating: ★★☆☆

Scallop and Ginger Skewers

Servings: 4

Preparation time: 20 minutes

Cooking time: 8 minutes

Ingredients:

- 24 large scallops
- 2 tablespoons soy sauce
- 1 tablespoon grated ginger
- 2 tablespoons sesame oil
- 1 green onion, finely sliced
- Wooden skewers, soaked in water

Directions:

1. In a bowl, mix soy sauce, sesame oil, and grated ginger.

2. Thread three scallops onto each skewer and brush them

with the soy ginger sauce.

3. Preheat a grill or grill pan over medium-high heat.

4. Grill the scallop skewers, turning occasionally, until opaque and slightly charred, about 2-3 minutes per side.

5. Sprinkle with green onions before serving.

Per serving: Calories: 200, Carbs: 5g, Fiber: 0g, Sugars: 0g, Protein: 18g, Saturated fat: 1g, Unsaturated fat: 9g

Difficulty rating: ★★☆☆

Garlic Butter Baked Cod

Servings: 4

Preparation time: 5 minutes

Cooking time: 15 minutes

Ingredients:

- 4 cod fillets (6 ounces each)
- 3 tablespoons butter, melted
- 4 cloves garlic, minced
- 1 tablespoon fresh parsley, chopped
- Juice of 1 lemon
- Salt and pepper to taste

Directions:

1. Preheat your oven to 400°F (200°C).

2. Place cod fillets in a baking dish.

3. In a small bowl, mix melted butter, garlic, parsley, and lemon juice. Season with salt and pepper.

4. Pour the garlic butter mixture over the cod fillets.

5. Bake in the preheated oven for about 15 minutes, or until fish flakes easily with a fork.

6. Serve immediately, spooning extra sauce from the dish over the fillets.

Per serving: Calories: 220, Carbs: 2g, Fiber: 0g, Sugars: 0g, Protein: 31g, Saturated fat: 5g, Unsaturated fat: 7g

Difficulty rating: ★☆☆☆☆

Mediterranean Tuna Salad

Servings: 4

Preparation time: 10 minutes

Cooking time: 0 minutes

Ingredients:

- 2 cans of tuna in olive oil, drained
- 1 cup cherry tomatoes, halved
- 1 cucumber, diced
- 1/2 red onion, thinly sliced
- 1/4 cup kalamata olives, pitted and halved
- 1/4 cup feta cheese, crumbled
- Juice of 1 lemon
- 2 tablespoons fresh basil, chopped
- Salt and pepper to taste

Directions:

1. In a large bowl, combine tuna, cherry tomatoes, cucumber, red onion, and kalamata olives.

2. Add lemon juice and toss to combine.

3. Gently fold in feta cheese and basil. Season with salt and pepper to taste.

4. Serve immediately or chill in the refrigerator for an hour to enhance flavors.

Per serving: Calories: 250, Carbs: 10g, Fiber: 2g, Sugars: 4g, Protein: 25g, Saturated fat: 3g, Unsaturated fat: 12g

Difficulty rating: ★☆☆☆☆

Lemon Garlic Scallops

Servings: 4

Preparation time: 5 minutes

Cooking time: 5 minutes

Ingredients:

- 1 lb scallops
- 2 tablespoons olive oil
- 3 cloves garlic, minced
- Juice of 1 lemon
- Salt and pepper to taste
- 2 tablespoons fresh parsley, chopped

Directions:

1. Heat olive oil in a large skillet over medium-high heat.

2. Add garlic and sauté for 1 minute until fragrant.

3. Add scallops to the skillet, season with salt and pepper, and cook for about 2 minutes on each side or until golden and translucent.

4. Remove from heat, drizzle with lemon juice, and garnish with parsley.

5. Serve immediately.

Per serving: Calories: 200, Carbs: 5g, Fiber: 0g, Sugars: 0g, Protein: 20g, Saturated fat: 1g, Unsaturated fat: 9g

Difficulty rating: ★★☆☆☆

Cilantro Lime Chicken

Servings: 4

Preparation time: 10 minutes

Cooking time: 15 minutes

Ingredients:

- 4 boneless, skinless chicken breasts
- 2 tablespoons olive oil
- Juice and zest of 2 limes
- 1/4 cup fresh cilantro, chopped
- 2 garlic cloves, minced
- 1 teaspoon honey
- Salt and pepper to taste

Directions:

1. In a bowl, whisk together olive oil, lime juice and zest, cilantro, garlic, and honey. Season with salt and pepper.

2. Place chicken breasts in the marinade and let sit for at least 30 minutes in the refrigerator.

3. Heat a grill or skillet over medium-high heat. Cook the chicken for about 7 minutes on each side, or until fully cooked and juices run clear.

4. Serve garnished with extra cilantro and lime wedges.

Per serving: Calories: 220, Carbs: 4g, Fiber: 0g, Sugars: 1g, Protein: 26g, Saturated fat: 2g, Unsaturated fat: 7g

Difficulty rating: ★☆☆☆☆

Quinoa Tabbouleh

Servings: 4

Preparation time: 15 minutes

Cooking time: 15 minutes

Ingredients:

- 1 cup quinoa, rinsed
- 2 cups water
- 1 cucumber, diced
- 2 medium tomatoes, diced
- 1/2 cup fresh parsley, finely chopped
- 1/4 cup fresh mint, finely chopped
- Juice of 1 lemon
- 3 tablespoons olive oil
- Salt and pepper to taste

Directions:

1. In a medium saucepan, bring water to a boil. Add quinoa and reduce heat to low. Cover and simmer for 15 minutes, or until water is absorbed.

2. Fluff quinoa with a fork and allow to cool.

3. In a large bowl, combine cooled quinoa, cucumber, tomatoes, parsley, and mint.

4. Dress with lemon juice and olive oil. Season with salt and pepper.

5. Chill in the refrigerator for at least one hour before serving to allow flavors to meld.

Per serving: Calories: 250, Carbs: 27g, Fiber: 4g, Sugars: 3g, Protein: 6g, Saturated fat: 1g, Unsaturated fat: 10g

Difficulty rating: ★★☆☆☆

Ginger Turmeric Salmon

Servings: 4

Preparation time: 10 minutes

Cooking time: 20 minutes

Ingredients:

- 4 salmon fillets (6 ounces each)
- 2 tablespoons olive oil
- 1 tablespoon freshly grated ginger
- 1 teaspoon turmeric
- 1 garlic clove, minced
- Salt and pepper to taste
- Lemon slices, for serving

Directions:

1. Preheat your oven to 375°F (190°C).

2. In a small bowl, mix olive oil, ginger, turmeric, and garlic. Season the mixture with salt and pepper.

3. Place salmon fillets on a baking sheet lined with parchment paper. Spread the ginger-turmeric mixture evenly over the fillets.

4. Bake in the preheated oven for about 15-20 minutes, or until salmon is cooked through and flakes easily with a fork.

5. Serve with fresh lemon slices.

Per serving: Calories: 300, Carbs: 2g, Fiber: 0.5g, Sugars: 0g, Protein: 23g, Saturated fat: 3g, Unsaturated fat: 13g

Difficulty rating: ★★☆☆☆

Avocado and Spinach Smoothie

Servings: 2

Preparation time: 5 minutes

Cooking time: 0 minutes

Ingredients:

- 1 ripe avocado, peeled and pitted
- 1 cup fresh spinach leaves
- 1 banana
- 1/2 cup unsweetened almond milk
- 1 tablespoon chia seeds
- Juice of 1/2 a lemon

Directions:

1. Place all ingredients in a blender.

2. Blend on high until smooth and creamy.

3. Serve immediately, garnished with a sprinkle of chia seeds if desired.

Per serving: Calories: 250, Carbs: 27g, Fiber: 9g, Sugars

: 10g, Protein: 4g, Saturated fat: 2g, Unsaturated fat: 15g

Difficulty rating: ★☆☆☆☆

Roasted Pepper and Hummus Wrap

Servings: 4

Preparation time: 10 minutes

Cooking time: 15 minutes

Ingredients:

- 4 whole wheat tortillas
- 1 cup hummus
- 2 bell peppers, sliced and roasted
- 1/2 red onion, thinly sliced
- 1/4 cup feta cheese, crumbled
- 1/4 cup fresh basil leaves

Directions:

1. Spread each tortilla with a layer of hummus.

2. Top with roasted bell peppers, red onion, feta cheese, and basil.

3. Roll up the tortillas tightly.

4. Serve immediately or grill for 2-3 minutes on each side if desired.

Per serving: Calories: 290, Carbs: 40g, Fiber: 7g, Sugars: 5g, Protein: 10g, Saturated fat: 3g, Unsaturated fat: 7g

Difficulty rating: ★☆☆☆☆

Spicy Bean and Tomato Stew

Servings: 4

Preparation time: 10 minutes

Cooking time: 20 minutes

Ingredients:

- 2 cans of mixed beans, drained and rinsed
- 1 large can diced tomatoes
- 1 onion, chopped
- 2 garlic cloves, minced
- 1 teaspoon cumin
- 1 teaspoon chili powder
- 2 tablespoons olive oil
- Salt and pepper to taste
- Fresh cilantro, for garnish

Directions:

1. Heat olive oil in a large pot over medium heat.

2. Add onion and garlic, sauté until soft.

3. Stir in cumin and chili powder, cooking for 1 minute until fragrant.

4. Add beans and tomatoes. Simmer for 15-20 minutes.

5. Season with salt and pepper.

6. Serve hot, garnished with fresh cilantro.

Per serving: Calories: 220, Carbs: 35g, Fiber: 9g, Sugars: 6g, Protein: 11g, Saturated fat: 1g, Unsaturated fat: 7g

Difficulty rating: ★☆☆☆☆

Spicy Grilled Shrimp Skewers

Servings: 4

Preparation time: 10 minutes (plus 30 minutes for marinating)

Cooking time: 5 minutes

Ingredients:

- 1 lb large shrimp, peeled and deveined
- 2 tablespoons olive oil
- 1 teaspoon smoked paprika
- 1/2 teaspoon red pepper flakes
- Juice of 1 lime
- Salt and pepper to taste
- Fresh cilantro, for garnish

Directions:

1. In a bowl, combine olive oil, smoked paprika, red pepper flakes, lime juice, salt, and pepper.

2. Add shrimp and toss to coat. Marinate in the refrigerator for 30 minutes.

3. Thread shrimp onto skewers.

4. Preheat grill to high heat and grill shrimp skewers for 2-3 minutes on each side, or until shrimp are pink and cooked through.

5. Garnish with cilantro and serve immediately.

Per serving: Calories: 180, Carbs: 2g, Fiber: 0g, Sugars: 0g, Protein: 24g, Saturated fat: 1g, Unsaturated fat: 7g

Difficulty rating: ★☆☆☆☆

Baked Lemon Pepper Tilapia

Servings: 4

Preparation time: 5 minutes

Cooking time: 15 minutes

Ingredients:

- 4 tilapia fillets
- Juice of 1 lemon
- 1 teaspoon black pepper
- 2 tablespoons olive oil
- Salt to taste
- Lemon slices, for garnish

Directions:

1. Preheat oven to 400°F (200°C).

2. Place tilapia fillets on a baking sheet. Drizzle with olive oil and lemon juice. Season with black pepper and salt.

3. Bake for 12-15 minutes or until fish is flaky and cooked through.

4. Serve immediately, garnished with lemon slices.

Per serving: Calories: 180, Carbs: 1g, Fiber: 0g, Sugars: 0g, Protein: 23g, Saturated fat: 2g, Unsaturated fat: 10g

Difficulty rating: ★☆☆☆☆

Zesty Carrot and Ginger Soup

Servings: 4

Preparation time: 10 minutes

Cooking time: 30 minutes

Ingredients:

- 1 lb carrots, peeled and chopped
- 4 cups vegetable broth
- 1 onion, chopped
- 2 tablespoons grated ginger
- 1 tablespoon olive oil
- Salt and pepper to taste
- Greek yogurt for serving (optional)

Directions:

1. Heat olive oil in a large pot over medium heat. Add onion and ginger, cook until onion is translucent.

2. Add carrots and vegetable broth. Bring to a boil, then simmer for 30 minutes until carrots are tender.

3. Blend the soup using an immersion blender until smooth.

4. Season with salt and pepper.

5. Serve hot, topped with a dollop of Greek yogurt if desired.

Per serving: Calories: 120, Carbs: 18g, Fiber: 5g, Sugars: 9g, Protein: 2g, Saturated fat: 1g, Unsaturated fat: 4g

Difficulty rating: ★☆☆☆☆

Natural Sweets

Cinnamon Apple Crisp

Servings: 6

Preparation time: 15 minutes

Cooking time: 45 minutes

Ingredients:

- 4 large apples, peeled, cored, and sliced
- 1/4 cup maple syrup
- 1 tsp ground cinnamon
- 1/2 cup rolled oats
- 1/4 cup almond flour
- 1/4 cup chopped walnuts
- 1/4 cup coconut oil, melted
- 1/2 tsp vanilla extract

Directions:

1. Preheat oven to 350°F (175°C).

2. Toss apple slices with 2 tablespoons of maple syrup and cinnamon. Place in a baking dish.

3. Mix oats, almond flour, walnuts, remaining maple syrup, coconut oil, and vanilla to form the topping. Spread over the apples.

4. Bake for 45 minutes until topping is golden and apples are tender.

5. Serve warm, optionally with a dollop of Greek yogurt.

Per serving: Calories: 290, Carbs: 38g, Fiber: 6g, Sugars: 24g, Protein: 4g, Saturated fat: 8g, Unsaturated fat: 5g

Difficulty rating: ★★☆☆☆

Chocolate Avocado Mousse

Servings: 4

Preparation time: 10 minutes

Cooking time: 0 minutes

Ingredients:

- 2 ripe avocados, peeled and pitted
- 1/4 cup cocoa powder
- 1/4 cup honey
- 1/2 cup coconut milk
- 1 tsp vanilla extract

Directions:

1. Combine all ingredients in a blender. Blend until smooth.

2. Divide the mousse into serving dishes and refrigerate for at least 1 hour.

3. Garnish with fresh berries or a sprinkle of chia seeds before serving.

Per serving: Calories: 250, Carbs: 35g, Fiber: 7g, Sugars: 23g, Protein: 3g, Saturated fat: 7g, Unsaturated fat: 10g

Difficulty rating: ★☆☆☆☆

Ginger Spiced Banana Bread

Servings: 10

Preparation time: 15 minutes

Cooking time: 1 hour

Ingredients:

- 3 ripe bananas, mashed
- 1/3 cup melted coconut oil
- 1/2 cup date sugar
- 1 egg, beaten
- 1 tsp vanilla extract
- 1 tsp baking soda
- Pinch of salt
- 1 1/2 cups whole wheat flour
- 1/2 tsp ground ginger
- 1/2 tsp ground cinnamon

Directions:

1. Preheat oven to 350°F (175°C). Grease a 9x5 inch loaf pan.

2. In a large bowl, stir together bananas, coconut oil, date sugar, egg, and vanilla.

3. Sprinkle baking soda and salt over the mixture, then add flour, ginger, and cinnamon. Stir just to blend.

4. Pour batter into the prepared loaf pan. Bake for 60 minutes, or until a toothpick inserted into the center comes out clean.

5. Let bread cool in the pan for 10 minutes, then turn out onto a wire rack to cool completely.

Per serving: Calories: 230, Carbs: 35g, Fiber: 4g, Sugars: 15g, Protein: 4g, Saturated fat: 6g, Unsaturated fat: 2g

Difficulty rating: ★★☆☆☆

Honey Glazed Blueberry Muffins

Servings: 12 muffins

Preparation time: 15 minutes

Cooking time: 25 minutes

Ingredients:

- 2 cups whole wheat flour
- 1 tsp baking powder
- 1/2 tsp baking soda
- 1/4 tsp salt
- 1/2 cup unsweetened applesauce
- 3/4 cup honey
- 1 egg
- 1 tsp vanilla extract
- 1 cup fresh blueberries
- 1/2 tsp lemon zest

Directions:

1. Preheat oven to 350°F (175°C). Line a muffin tin with paper liners.

2. In a bowl, mix together flour, baking powder, baking soda, and salt.

3. In another bowl, whisk together applesauce, honey, egg, and vanilla.

4. Combine wet and dry ingredients until just mixed. Fold in blueberries and lemon zest.

5. Divide batter evenly among muffin cups. Bake for 25 minutes or until a toothpick inserted into the center comes out clean.

6. Serve warm or let cool on a wire rack.

Per serving: Calories: 180, Carbs: 37g, Fiber: 3g, Sugars: 20g, Protein: 3g, Saturated fat: 0.5g, Unsaturated fat: 1g

Difficulty rating: ★☆☆☆☆

Pear and Walnut Crumble

Servings: 6

Preparation time: 15 minutes

Cooking time: 30 minutes

Ingredients:

- 4 ripe pears, peeled, cored, and sliced
- 1/3 cup maple syrup
- 1 teaspoon ground cinnamon
- 1 cup rolled oats
- 1/2 cup walnuts, chopped
- 1/4 cup almond flour
- 1/4 cup coconut oil, softened

Directions:

1. Preheat the oven to 375°F (190°C).

2. Toss the pear slices with 2 tablespoons of maple syrup and cinnamon, then spread them into a baking dish.

3. In a bowl, combine oats, walnuts, almond flour, remaining maple syrup, and coconut oil until the mixture resembles coarse crumbs.

4. Sprinkle the crumble mixture over the pears.

5. Bake for 30 minutes, or until the topping is golden and the pears are tender.

6. Serve warm.

Per serving: Calories: 300, Carbs: 38g, Fiber: 6g, Sugars: 20g, Protein: 4g, Saturated fat: 6g, Unsaturated fat: 4g

Difficulty rating: ★★☆☆☆

Carrot Cake Energy Balls

Servings: 12 balls

Preparation time: 20 minutes

Cooking time: 0 minutes

Ingredients:

- 1 cup shredded carrots
- 1 cup dates, pitted
- 1/2 cup rolled oats
- 1/2 cup unsweetened shredded coconut
- 1/4 cup walnuts, finely chopped
- 1 teaspoon vanilla extract
- 1 teaspoon ground cinnamon

Directions:

1. Place all ingredients in a food processor and pulse until well combined.

2. Roll the mixture into small balls, about the size of a walnut.

3. Refrigerate for at least 30 minutes before serving to allow the flavors to meld.

4. Store in an airtight container in the refrigerator.

Per serving: Calories: 120, Carbs: 18g, Fiber: 3g, Sugars: 12g, Protein: 2g, Saturated fat: 2g, Unsaturated fat: 2g

Difficulty rating: ★☆☆☆☆

Coconut Yogurt Parfait

Servings: 4

Preparation time: 10 minutes

Cooking time: 0 minutes

Ingredients:

- 2 cups unsweetened coconut yogurt
- 1/2 cup homemade granola (use maple syrup for sweetening)
- 1 cup mixed berries (strawberries, blueberries, raspberries)
- 1 tablespoon honey (optional)

Directions:

1. In serving glasses, layer coconut yogurt, a spoonful of granola, and a layer of mixed berries.

2. Repeat the layers until the glasses are filled.

3. Drizzle with honey if desired and serve immediately.

Per serving: Calories: 180, Carbs: 25g, Fiber: 3g, Sugars: 15g, Protein: 6g, Saturated fat: 4g, Unsaturated fat: 1g

Difficulty rating: ★☆☆☆☆

Spiced Ginger Tea

Servings: 4

Preparation time: 5 minutes

Cooking time: 10 minutes

Ingredients:

- 4 cups water
- 2 inches fresh ginger, thinly sliced
- 2 cinnamon sticks
- 2 tablespoons honey
- Juice of 1 lemon

Directions:

1. In a saucepan, bring water, ginger, and cinnamon sticks to a boil.

2. Reduce heat and simmer for 10 minutes.

3. Strain the tea into cups, stir in honey and lemon juice, and serve.

Per serving: Calories: 40, Carbs: 10g, Fiber: 0g, Sugars: 9g, Protein: 0g, Saturated fat: 0g, Unsaturated fat: 0g

Difficulty rating: ★☆☆☆☆

Almond and Date Truffles

Servings: 12 truffles

Preparation time: 15 minutes

Cooking time: 0 minutes

Ingredients:

- 1 cup almonds
- 1 cup medjool dates, pitted
- 1/4 cup cocoa powder
- 1 teaspoon vanilla extract
- A pinch of sea salt
- Unsweetened cocoa powder, for dusting

Directions:

1. In a food processor, combine almonds and dates until finely chopped and sticky.

2. Add cocoa powder, vanilla extract, and sea salt. Process until the mixture forms a dough-like consistency.

3. Roll the mixture into small balls, then dust with cocoa powder.

4. Chill in the refrigerator for at least an hour before serving.

Per serving: Calories: 150, Carbs: 18g, Fiber: 3g, Sugars: 14g, Protein: 3g, Saturated fat: 0.5g, Unsaturated fat: 3g

Difficulty rating: ★★☆☆☆

Baked Pears with Walnuts and Honey

Servings: 4

Preparation time: 10 minutes

Cooking time: 25 minutes

Ingredients:

- 4 pears, halved and cored
- 1/4 cup walnuts, chopped
- 4 teaspoons honey
- 1/2 teaspoon ground cinnamon

Directions:

1. Preheat the oven to 350°F (175°C).

2. Place pear halves on a baking sheet, cut side up.

3. Sprinkle with cinnamon, top with walnuts, and drizzle with honey.

4. Bake for 25 minutes, or until pears are tender and topping is golden.

5. Serve warm.

Per serving: Calories: 200, Carbs: 38g, Fiber: 6g, Sugars: 28g, Protein: 2g, Saturated fat: 0g, Unsaturated fat: 2g

Difficulty rating: ★☆☆☆☆

Vanilla Chia Pudding with Fresh Berries

Servings: 4

Preparation time: 10 minutes (plus chilling)

Cooking time: 0 minutes

Ingredients:

- 1/4 cup chia seeds
- 1 cup unsweetened almond milk
- 1 teaspoon vanilla extract
- 2 tablespoons maple syrup
- 1 cup mixed fresh berries (blueberries, raspberries, strawberries)
- Mint leaves for garnish (optional)

Directions:

1. In a mixing bowl, combine chia seeds, almond milk, vanilla extract, and maple syrup. Stir well until the mixture begins to thicken.

2. Cover the bowl and refrigerate for at least 2 hours, or overnight, until it reaches a pudding-like consistency.

3. To serve, spoon the chia pudding into bowls or glasses and top with fresh berries.

4. Garnish with mint leaves if desired.

Per serving: Calories: 150, Carbs: 20g, Fiber: 5g, Sugars: 12g, Protein: 3g, Saturated fat: 0.5g, Unsaturated fat: 2g

Difficulty rating: ★☆☆☆☆

Apple Cinnamon Baked Oatmeal

Servings: 6

Preparation time: 15 minutes

Cooking time: 35 minutes

Ingredients:

- 2 cups rolled oats
- 1 teaspoon baking powder
- 1 1/2 teaspoons ground cinnamon
- 1/4 teaspoon salt
- 1 apple, peeled, cored, and diced
- 1/4 cup chopped walnuts
- 2 cups unsweetened almond milk
- 1/4 cup honey
- 1 large egg
- 2 teaspoons vanilla extract

Directions:

1. Preheat the oven to 375°F (190°C). Grease an 8x8 inch baking dish.

2. In a large bowl, mix together oats, baking powder, cinnamon, and salt.

3. Stir in diced apple and walnuts.

4. In another bowl, whisk together almond milk, honey, egg, and vanilla extract.

5. Pour the liquid ingredients over the oat mixture and stir until combined.

6. Transfer the mixture to the prepared baking dish and spread evenly.

7. Bake in the preheated oven for 35 minutes, or until the top is golden and the oats are set.

8. Serve warm, optionally topped with additional honey or fresh fruit.

Per serving: Calories: 230, Carbs: 38g, Fiber: 5g, Sugars: 17g, Protein: 6g, Saturated fat: 0.5g, Unsaturated fat: 3g

Difficulty rating: ★★☆☆☆

Simple Sauces & Dressings

Basil and Lemon Vinaigrette

Servings: 4

Preparation time: 5 minutes

Cooking time: 0 minutes

Ingredients:

- 1/4 cup olive oil
- Juice and zest of 1 lemon
- 1/4 cup fresh basil leaves, finely chopped
- 1 clove garlic, minced
- Salt and pepper to taste

Directions:

1. In a small bowl, whisk together olive oil, lemon juice, lemon zest, chopped basil, and minced garlic.

2. Season with salt and pepper to taste.

3. Serve drizzled over fresh salads or grilled vegetables.

Per serving: Calories: 120, Carbs: 1g, Fiber: 0g, Sugars: 0g, Protein: 0g, Saturated fat: 2g, Unsaturated fat: 10g

Difficulty rating: ★☆☆☆☆

Rosemary-Garlic Infused Olive Oil

Servings: 4

Preparation time: 5 minutes

Cooking time: 10 minutes

Ingredients:

- 1/2 cup olive oil
- 3 cloves garlic, thinly sliced
- 2 sprigs fresh rosemary

Directions:

1. Combine olive oil, garlic slices, and rosemary sprigs in a small saucepan.

2. Gently heat on low for 10 minutes, careful not to let the garlic brown.

3. Remove from heat and let cool. Strain the oil and discard the solids.

4. Use as a finishing oil for meats or roasted vegetables.

Per serving: Calories: 120, Carbs: 0g, Fiber: 0g, Sugars: 0g, Protein: 0g, Saturated fat: 2g, Unsaturated fat: 10g

Difficulty rating: ★☆☆☆☆

Tangy Orange and Thyme Dressing

Servings: 4

Preparation time: 5 minutes

Cooking time: 0 minutes

Ingredients:

- 1/4 cup olive oil
- Juice and zest of 1 orange
- 1 tablespoon fresh thyme leaves
- 1 teaspoon honey
- Salt and pepper to taste

Directions:

1. In a bowl, whisk together olive oil, orange juice, orange zest, thyme leaves, and honey.

2. Season with salt and pepper to taste.

3. Ideal for dressing leafy green salads or drizzling over grilled chicken.

Per serving: Calories: 120, Carbs: 3g, Fiber: 0g, Sugars: 2g, Protein: 0g, Saturated fat: 2g, Unsaturated fat: 10g

Difficulty rating: ★☆☆☆☆

Cilantro Lime Dressing

Servings: 4

Preparation time: 5 minutes

Cooking time: 0 minutes

Ingredients:

- 1/4 cup olive oil
- Juice and zest of 2 limes
- 1/4 cup fresh cilantro, chopped
- 1 clove garlic, minced
- 1 teaspoon honey
- Salt and pepper to taste

Directions:

1. In a small bowl, whisk together olive oil, lime juice, lime zest, chopped cilantro, minced garlic, and honey.

2. Season with salt and pepper to taste.

3. Serve with tacos, fajitas, or as a salad dressing.

Per serving: Calories: 120, Carbs: 4g, Fiber: 0g, Sugars: 3g, Protein: 0g, Saturated fat: 2g, Unsaturated fat: 10g

Difficulty rating: ★☆☆☆☆

Mint Yogurt Sauce

Servings: 4

Preparation time: 5 minutes

Cooking time: 0 minutes

Ingredients:

- 1 cup plain Greek yogurt
- 1/4 cup fresh mint, finely chopped
- Juice of 1 lemon
- 1 clove garlic, minced
- Salt and pepper to taste

Directions:

1. In a bowl, combine Greek yogurt, chopped mint, lemon juice, and minced garlic.

2. Season with salt and pepper to taste.

3. Chill before serving as a dip with vegetables or as a sauce for grilled lamb.

Nutritional

 value per serving: Calories: 70, Carbs: 4g, Fiber: 0g, Sugars: 3g, Protein: 6g, Saturated fat: 0.5g, Unsaturated fat: 0g

Difficulty rating: ★☆☆☆

Creamy Avocado Dressing

Servings: 4

Preparation time: 5 minutes

Cooking time: 0 minutes

Ingredients:

- 1 ripe avocado, peeled and pitted
- 1/4 cup olive oil
- Juice of 1 lime
- 1 clove garlic, minced
- Salt and pepper to taste

Directions:

1. In a blender, combine avocado, olive oil, lime juice, and garlic.

2. Blend until smooth. Season with salt and pepper to taste.

3. Serve as a creamy dressing for salads or as a dip for chips and veggies.

Per serving: Calories: 150, Carbs: 8g, Fiber: 4g, Sugars: 1g, Protein: 2g, Saturated fat: 2g, Unsaturated fat: 10g

Difficulty rating: ★☆☆☆

Honey Mustard Vinaigrette

Servings: 4

Preparation time: 5 minutes

Cooking time: 0 minutes

Ingredients:

- 1/4 cup olive oil
- 2 tablespoons apple cider vinegar
- 1 tablespoon honey
- 1 tablespoon Dijon mustard
- Salt and pepper to taste

Directions:

1. In a small bowl, whisk together olive oil, apple cider vinegar, honey, and Dijon mustard.

2. Season with salt and pepper to taste.

3. Perfect for dressing salads or as a marinade for chicken.

Per serving: Calories: 140, Carbs: 5g, Fiber: 0g, Sugars: 4g, Protein: 0g, Saturated fat: 2g, Unsaturated fat: 10g

Difficulty rating: ★☆☆☆☆

Garlic Herb Marinade

Servings: 4

Preparation time: 5 minutes

Cooking time: 0 minutes

Ingredients:

- 1/3 cup olive oil
- 3 cloves garlic, minced
- 1 tablespoon chopped fresh rosemary
- 1 tablespoon chopped fresh thyme
- Juice of 1 lemon
- Salt and pepper to taste

Directions:

1. In a bowl, combine olive oil, minced garlic, chopped rosemary, chopped thyme, and lemon juice.

2. Season with salt and pepper to taste.

3. Use as a marinade for meats or vegetables before grilling or roasting.

Per serving: Calories: 120, Carbs: 2g, Fiber: 0g, Sugars: 0g, Protein: 0g, Saturated fat: 2g, Unsaturated fat: 10g

Difficulty rating: ★☆☆☆☆

Balsamic Fig Dressing

Servings: 4

Preparation time: 5 minutes

Cooking time: 0 minutes

Ingredients:

- 1/4 cup olive oil
- 2 tablespoons balsamic vinegar
- 3 fresh figs, stemmed and quartered
- 1 teaspoon Dijon mustard
- 1 clove garlic, minced
- Salt and pepper to taste

Directions:

1. In a blender, combine olive oil, balsamic vinegar, figs, Dijon mustard, and minced garlic.

2. Blend until smooth and creamy. Season with salt and pepper to taste.

3. Serve as a unique dressing for green salads or drizzle over roasted vegetables.

Per serving: Calories: 150, Carbs: 10g, Fiber: 1g, Sugars: 8g, Protein: 0g, Saturated fat: 2g, Unsaturated fat: 10g

Difficulty rating: ★☆☆☆☆

Lemon Basil Pesto

Servings: 4

Preparation time: 10 minutes

Cooking time: 0 minutes

Ingredients:

- 1 cup fresh basil leaves
- 1/3 cup olive oil
- 1/4 cup pine nuts
- 2 tablespoons lemon juice
- 2 cloves garlic
- Salt and pepper to taste
- Grated Parmesan cheese (optional)

Directions:

1. In a food processor, combine basil leaves, olive oil, pine nuts, lemon juice, and garlic.

2. Process until smooth, scraping down the sides as needed.

3. Season with salt and pepper, and mix in Parmesan cheese if desired.

4. Use as a sauce for pasta, a spread for sandwiches, or a garnish for grilled meats.

Per serving: Calories: 220, Carbs: 3g, Fiber: 1g, Sugars: 1g, Protein: 2g, Saturated fat: 2g, Unsaturated fat: 18g

Difficulty rating: ★★☆☆☆

Spicy Avocado Cilantro Lime Dressing

Servings: 4

Preparation time: 5 minutes

Cooking time: 0 minutes

Ingredients:

- 1 ripe avocado
- 1/4 cup fresh cilantro, chopped
- Juice of 2 limes
- 1/2 teaspoon red pepper flakes
- 1/4 cup olive oil
- Salt and pepper to taste

Directions:

1. In a blender, combine avocado, cilantro, lime juice, red pepper flakes, and olive oil.

2. Blend until smooth and creamy. Season with salt and pepper to taste.

3. Ideal for drizzling over tacos, adding to bowls, or as a dip for fresh veggies.

Per serving: Calories: 190, Carbs: 6g, Fiber: 3g, Sugars: 1g, Protein: 1g, Saturated fat: 3g, Unsaturated fat: 14g

Difficulty rating: ★☆☆☆☆

Roasted Garlic and Herb Aioli

Servings: 4

Preparation time: 5 minutes (plus time for roasting garlic)

Cooking time: 30 minutes (for roasting garlic)

Ingredients:

- 1 whole garlic bulb
- 1/2 cup olive oil
- 1 egg yolk
- 1 tablespoon lemon juice
- 1 tablespoon fresh parsley, chopped
- Salt and pepper to taste

Directions:

1. Preheat oven to 400°F (200°C). Cut the top off the garlic bulb to expose cloves, drizzle with a bit of olive oil, and wrap in foil. Roast in the oven for about 30 minutes or until cloves are soft and golden.

2. Squeeze the roasted garlic cloves into a food processor. Add egg yolk, lemon juice, and remaining olive oil.

3. Blend until the mixture is smooth and creamy. Stir in chopped parsley, and season with salt and pepper.

4. Serve as a dip with vegetables, a spread for sandwiches, or a topping for grilled meats.

Per serving: Calories: 260, Carbs: 5g, Fiber: 0g, Sugars: 0g, Protein: 1g, Saturated fat: 4g, Unsaturated fat: 20g

Difficulty rating: ★★☆☆☆

Conclusion

As we draw to a close on this exploration of anti-inflammatory eating, I wish to share a more personal touch, a glimpse into the journey behind the recipes. Creating this book was more than a professional task; it was an emotional adventure filled with trials, triumphs, and the inevitable learning curve that accompanies innovation in the kitchen. Each page is imbued not only with my passion for healthy cooking but also with my desire to impart something genuinely valuable to you.

Your support is incredibly important to me. Every comment and reflection you share about this book guides my path as an author. Your feedback helps me evolve and improves the reading and cooking experience for others, illuminating the path to discovering the joys of anti-inflammatory cuisine.

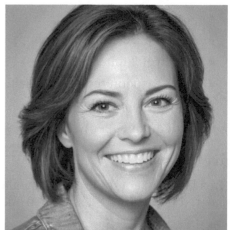

I realize that every review comes from someone with unique experiences and expectations, and I promise to consider each of your thoughts with care and gratitude. It is this dialogue, this connection between us, that enriches the book world.

Imagine me in my kitchen, surrounded by the very ingredients we've discussed, hands busily preparing dishes, with a smile, eager to share this passion with you. This scene, though intangible, encapsulates the essence of what I've strived to convey: a love for simple, wholesome, and delicious food. It is in these moments of creation and sharing that the true spirit of this cookbook is realized.

If the recipes and tips within these pages have added flavor and health to your table and life, I invite you to access a special bonus—the "Anti-Inflammatory Plant-Based Recipe Booklet." Instead of a traditional download link, please scan the QR code below to receive this additional gift. Your engagement is powerful, and every expression about this book strengthens the bond between us, fostering a shared journey of culinary discovery and growth.

Please scan the QR code below to receive your bonus recipe booklet:

Thank you from the bottom of my heart for joining me on this journey, for every moment you've spent exploring the pages I've crafted with care for you.

28 DAY MEAL PLAN

WEEK 1

Day	Breakfast	Lunch	Dinner	Snacks
1	Almond Butter and Banana Toast (p. 25)	Sweet Potato and Ginger Soup (p. 41)	Rosemary Lemon Chicken Skewers (p. 73)	Carrot Sticks with Almond Butter Dip (p. 35)
2	Spinach and Feta Omelette (p. 25)	Tomato and White Bean Soup (p. 43)	Grilled Mackerel with Orange and Fennel (p. 83)	Kale Chips with Nutritional Yeast (p. 36)
3	Turmeric Oatmeal with Blueberries (p. 26)	Vegetable Minestrone (p. 46)	Turmeric Ginger Turkey Burgers (p. 73)	Mixed Berry Energy Bites (p. 36)
4	Avocado and Egg Breakfast Bowl (p. 26)	Lentil and Spinach Soup (p. 45)	Cauliflower Steak with Turmeric Quinoa (p. 61)	Spicy Roasted Chickpeas (p. 37)
5	Ginger Pear Smoothie Bowl (p. 27)	Spicy Black Bean Soup (p. 46)	Lemon Herb Poached Salmon (p. 83)	Avocado Lime Hummus (p. 37)
6	Quinoa Breakfast Bowl with Avocado (p. 27)	Carrot and Coriander Soup (p. 47)	Beef and Barley Stew with Carrots (p. 44)	Pumpkin Spice Granola (p. 38)
7	Pumpkin Spice Oatmeal (p. 30)	Chicken Noodle Soup with Turmeric (p. 49)	Broccoli and Almond Soup (p. 48)	Beetroot and Walnut Dip (p. 38)

WEEK 2

Day	Breakfast	Lunch	Dinner	Snack
8	Quinoa Breakfast Bowl with Avocado (p. 27)	Creamy Butternut Squash Soup (p. 44)	Baked Sardines with Lemon and Herbs (p. 84)	Pumpkin Spice Granola (p. 38)
9	Berry Almond Overnight Oats (p. 31)	Lemon Garlic Scallops (p. 87)	Turmeric Ginger Turkey Burgers (p. 73)	Mixed Berry Energy Bites (p. 36)
10	Chia Seed Pudding with Mixed Berries (p. 28)	Tomato and Turmeric Stew (p. 43)	Cauliflower Steak with Turmeric Quinoa (p. 61)	Spicy Roasted Chickpeas (p. 37)
11	Berry Almond Overnight Oats (p. 31)	Vegetable Minestrone (p. 46)	Lemon Herb Poached Salmon (p. 83)	Avocado Lime Hummus (p. 37)
12	Vegan Banana Pancakes (p. 32)	Lentil and Spinach Soup (p. 45)	Rosemary Lemon Chicken Skewers (p. 73)	Beetroot and Walnut Dip (p. 38)
13	Almond Butter Toast with Banana (p. 33)	Carrot and Ginger Soup (p. 41)	Mushroom and Thyme Stew (p. 47)	Carrot Sticks with Almond Butter Dip (p. 35)
14	Savory Quinoa Porridge with Avocado (p. 33)	Spicy Black Bean Soup (p. 46)	Chili-Lime Shrimp Tacos (p. 85)	Kale Chips with Nutritional Yeast (p. 36)

28 DAY MEAL PLAN

WEEK 3

Day	Breakfast	Lunch	Dinner	Snack
15	Quinoa Breakfast Bowl with Avocado (p. 27)	Creamy Butternut Squash Soup (p. 44)	Balsamic Glazed Pork Tenderloin (p. 74)	Pumpkin Spice Granola (p. 38)
16	Berry Almond Overnight Oats (p. 31)	Lemon Garlic Scallops (p. 87)	Cauliflower Steak with Turmeric Quinoa (p. 61)	Mixed Berry Energy Bites (p. 36)
17	Chia Seed Pudding with Mixed Berries (p. 28)	Tomato and Turmeric Stew (p. 43)	Rosemary Lemon Chicken Skewers (p. 73)	Spicy Roasted Chickpeas (p. 37)
18	Berry Almond Overnight Oats (p. 31)	Vegetable Minestrone (p. 46)	Lemon Herb Poached Salmon (p. 83)	Avocado Lime Hummus (p. 37)
19	Vegan Banana Pancakes (p. 32)	Lentil and Spinach Soup (p. 45)	Turmeric Ginger Turkey Burgers (p. 73)	Beetroot and Walnut Dip (p. 38)
20	Almond Butter Toast with Banana (p. 33)	Carrot and Ginger Soup (p. 41)	Mushroom and Thyme Stew (p. 47)	Carrot Sticks with Almond Butter Dip (p. 35)
21	Savory Quinoa Porridge with Avocado (p. 33)	Spicy Black Bean Soup (p. 46)	Chili-Lime Shrimp Tacos (p. 85)	Kale Chips with Nutritional Yeast (p. 36)

WEEK 4

Day	Breakfast	Lunch	Dinner	Snack
22	Pumpkin Spice Oatmeal (p. 30)	Chicken Noodle Soup with Turmeric (p. 49)	Balsamic Glazed Pork Tenderloin (p. 74)	Beetroot and Walnut Dip (p. 38)
23	Vegan Banana Pancakes (p. 32)	Creamy Butternut Squash Soup (p. 44)	Grilled Mackerel with Orange and Fennel (p. 83)	Kale Chips with Nutritional Yeast (p. 36)
24	Almond Butter Toast with Banana (p. 33)	Tomato and Turmeric Stew (p. 43)	Cauliflower Steak with Turmeric Quinoa (p. 61)	Mixed Berry Energy Bites (p. 36)
25	Savory Quinoa Porridge with Avocado (p. 33)	Vegetable Minestrone (p. 46)	Lemon Herb Poached Salmon (p. 83)	Pumpkin Spice Granola (p. 38)
26	Chia Seed Pudding with Mixed Berries (p. 28)	Lentil and Spinach Soup (p. 45)	Rosemary Lemon Chicken Skewers (p. 73)	Spicy Roasted Chickpeas (p. 37)
27	Berry Almond Overnight Oats (p. 31)	Carrot and Ginger Soup (p. 41)	Chili-Lime Shrimp Tacos (p. 85)	Avocado Lime Hummus (p. 37)
28	Quinoa and Berry Breakfast Cups (p. 34)	Spicy Black Bean Soup (p. 46)	Mushroom and Thyme Stew (p. 47)	Carrot Sticks with Almond Butter Dip (p. 35)

Conversion Chart

Volume Equivalents (Liquid)

US Standard	US Standard (oz.)	Metric (approximate)
2 tbsps.	1 fl. oz.	30 milliliter
¼ cup	2 fl. oz.	60 milliliter
½ cup	4 fl. oz.	120 milliliter
1 cup	8 fl. oz.	240 milliliter
1½ cups	12 fl. oz.	355 milliliter
2 cups or 1 pint	16 fl. oz.	475 milliliter
4 cups or 1 quart	32 fl. oz.	1 Liter
1 gallon	128 fl. oz.	4 Liter

Volume Equivalents (Dry)

US Standard	Metric (approximate)
⅛ tsp.	0.5 milliliter
¼ tsp.	1 milliliter
½ tsp.	2 milliliter
¾ tsp.	4 milliliter
1 tsp.	5 milliliter
1 tbsp.	15 milliliter
¼ cup	59 milliliter
⅓ cup	79 milliliter
½ cup	118 milliliter
⅔ cup	156 milliliter
¾ cup	177 milliliter
1 cup	235 milliliter
2 cups or 1 pint	475 milliliter
3 cups	700 milliliter
4 cups or 1 quart	1 Liter

Oven Temperatures

Fahrenheit (F)	Celsius (C) (approximate)
250 °F	120 °C
300 °F	150 °C
325 °F	165 °C
350 °F	180 °C
375 °F	190 °C
400 °F	200 °C
425 °F	220 °C
450 °F	230 °C

Weight Equivalents

US Standard	Metric (approximate)
1 tbsp.	15 g
½ oz.	15 g
1 oz.	30 g
2 oz.	60 g
4 oz.	115 g
8 oz.	225 g
12 oz.	340 g
16 oz. or 1 lb.	455 g

INDEX

Made in United States
Troutdale, OR
08/17/2024

22108041R00064